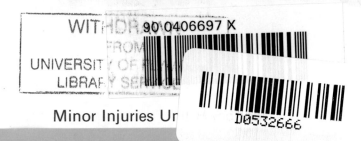

WITHDRAWN 90 0406697 X
FROM
UNIVERSITY OF
LIBRARY SERVICES

D0532666

Minor Injuries Un

TWENTY ONE DAY LOAN

This item is to be returned on
or before the date stamped below

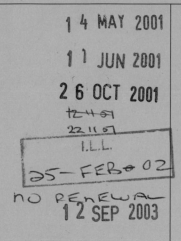

1 4 MAY 2001   2 9 JAN 2004

1 1 JUN 2001

2 6 OCT 2001

12-4-01

22-11-01

I.L.L.

25 - FEB - 02

no RENEWAL

1 2 SEP 2003

UNIVERSITY OF PLYMOUTH

PLYMOUTH LIBRARY

Tel: (01752) 232323
This item is available for the student loan period of 21 days
It is subject to recall if required by another reader
CHARGES WILL BE MADE FOR OVERDUE BOOKS

WIT
UNIVERSIT
LIBRAR

Minor Injuries Unit Handbook

A guide for A&E Senior House Officers, Emergency Nurse Practitioners and General Practitioners

Matthew Cooke MB FRCS FFAEM DipIMC RCS(Ed)

Senior Lecturer, Department of General Practice, University of Birmingham and City Hospital, Birmingham

Ellen Jones MRCP FFAEM

Consultant in Accident and Emergency Medicine, Birmingham Heartlands Hospital, Birmingham

Conor Kelly FRCS FFAEM

Consultant in Accident and Emergency Medicine, City Hospital, Birmingham

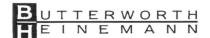

OXFORD BOSTON JOHANNESBURG MELBOURNE NEW DELHI SINGAPORE

Butterworth-Heinemann
Linacre House, Jordan Hill, Oxford OX2 8DP
225 Wildwood Avenue, Woburn, MA 01801-2041

A division of Reed Educational and Professional Publishing Ltd

A member of the Reed Elsevier plc group

First published 1998

© Reed Educational and Professional Publishing Ltd 1998

All rights reserved. No part of this publication may be reproduced in
any material form (including photocopying or storing in any medium by
electronic means and whether or not transiently or incidentally to some
other use of this publication) without the written permission of the
copyright holder except in accordance with the provisions of the Copyright,
Designs and Patents Act 1988 or under the terms of a licence issued by the
Copyright Licensing Agency Ltd, 90 Tottenham Court Road, London,
England W1P 9HE. Applications for the copyright holder's written
permission to reproduce any part of this publication should be addressed
to the publishers

British Library Cataloguing in Publication Data
Cooke, Matthew
  Minor injuries unit handbook
  1. Emergency medicine
  I. Title   II. Jones, Ellen   III. Kelly, Conor
  616'.025

ISBN 0 7506 3451 0

Library of Congress Cataloguing in Publication Data
  Minor injuries unit handbook : a guide for A&E senior house
  officers, emergency nurse practitioners, and general practitioners /
  Matthew Cooke, Ellen Jones, Conor Kelly.
  p. cm.
  Includes bibliographical references and index.
  ISBN 0 7506 3451 0
  1. Wounds and injuries.   2. Medical emergencies.   3. Hospitals–
  Emergency service.   I. Jones, Ellen, MB ChB.   II. Kelly, Conor.
  III. Title.
  [DNLM: 1. Wounds and Injuries – therapy handbooks.   2. Emergencies
  handbooks.   3. Emergency Treatment handbooks.   4. Accidents
  handbooks.   WO 39C773m]
  RD93.C68
  617.1 – dc21   98–26929 CIP

Data manipulation by David Gregson Associates, Beccles, Suffolk
Printed and bound in Great Britain by MPG Books, Bodmin, Cornwall

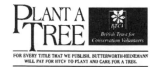

FOR EVERY TITLE THAT WE PUBLISH, BUTTERWORTH-HEINEMANN
WILL PAY FOR BTCV TO PLANT AND CARE FOR A TREE.

Contents

UNIVERSITY OF PLYMOUTH

Item No. 900406697X

Date 1 4 MAR 2000

Class No. 617.1 COO

Contl. No. ✓

LIBRARY SERVICES

Section 3	Medical conditions that present at minor injuries units

Section 4	**Managerial matters at minor injuries units**

Preface

The management of minor injuries and complaints can be difficult to learn: they do not fit speciality categories and are therefore not covered well in standard texts, little evidence is available on their management and while training we tend to concentrate on more serious conditions. However, many health professionals are dealing with emergencies in A&E departments, minor injury units, general practice and other settings. All need to be able to deal with the minor problems that are considered emergencies.

Minor conditions are often more difficult than the obvious life-threatening condition. It is important not to miss the unusual presentation of a serious condition or miss the more complex case. Many textbooks only briefly mention these minor cases. We have therefore written this book to help all those who deal with minor emergencies. The book will supplement the textbook of A&E medicine for the A&E Senior House Officer. It will add to the protocols of the Nurse Practitioner. It will assist the General Practitioner in the emergency centre.

We have based our text on evidence wherever possible. However, for many minor conditions, consensus is the best evidence. We have not listed all possible treatments or attempted to demonstrate all the variations in care. We supply what we believe to be an effective and safe method of care wherever it is practised.

We hope this book makes the stressful task of caring for emergencies easier, simpler and safer for all.

MWC
EJ
CK

Acknowledgements

To Heather, David and Rosaire for all their support during the writing of this book.

Section I

Wound care

Wound assessment

- Listen to what the patient says
- Take time to examine the wound and deeper structures
- Examine each structure in turn and document findings.

ASSESSMENT

1. History of injury
2. Mechanism
3. Possibility of foreign body
4. Risk of infection
5. Past history
   - tetanus immunization status
   - allergy
   - medication
6. Examination
   - wound
       site
       shape
       edges
   - foreign bodies/dirt
   - underlying structures
       tendons
       nerves
       vessels
       bone
       joint
7. Investigations
   - radiology – bone/joint injury
8. Foreign bodies
   - wound swabs
   - infected wounds.

INDICATION FOR REFERRAL

1. Suspicion of injury to deeper structures
2. Foreign bodies
3. Wounds too extensive for management in your setting.

(When to refer and to whom will depend on local practice.)

Wound cleaning

- Most important aspect of wound care
- For vigorous cleaning, analgesia/anaesthesia will be required.

PREPARATION

1. The surrounding area should be 'socially' clean
2. Use soap and water or degreasing agents
3. Washing under the tap is very effective for initial cleaning of wounds.

METHOD

1. Aseptic technique
2. Always wear gloves
3. For cleaning around the wound, use swab soaked in cleaning solution and held in forceps
4. For cleaning the wound, use gauze to remove clots, debris etc.
5. Use scrubbing brush/nail brush to remove ingrained dirt
6. Necrotic or adherent material may need excision
7. Irrigation with normal saline.

Caution – If the wound is not clean, leave it open and consider delayed primary closure.

Wound closure

KEY POINTS

- Thorough wound cleaning is essential
- If in doubt, leave wound open
- Some wounds are best left open, e.g. bites on hand
- Delayed primary closure may be preferred in wounds that are at high risk of developing infection.

PREPARATION

1. Ensure no underlying damage requiring specialist treatment
2. Ensure adequate light
3. Ensure adequate anaesthesia
4. Have help as required.

OPTIONS

1. Steristrips
2. Glue
3. Sutures.

Dressings

- There are many different types of products available, and most departments will have their own practice
- There are situations in which the wound may be left uncovered
- All wounds need thorough cleaning prior to dressing
- Give the patient the opportunity to wash.

OPTIONS

1. Sutured wounds
   - may be left uncovered
   - dry non-adherent dressings may be applied to protect wound from clothing etc.
2. Open wounds and partial thickness wounds, e.g. abrasions, burns, road rash
   - use paraffin impregnated gauze, e.g. Jelonet™, Bactigras™ or hydrocolloid, e.g. Granuflex™
3. Sloughy wounds
   - use e.g. Xerogel™, Kaltostat™
   - Scherisorb™
4. Necrotic wounds
   - use hydrocolloid, e.g. Granuflex™
   - may need surgical excision of dead tissue.

CAUTION

1. Do not let dressing dry out
2. If dry, the dressing may need to soaked off
3. When to redress will depend on the size and degree of infection of the wound. In a clean wound that is dry, it is often best to leave the dressing as long as possible.

Local anaesthesia

KEY POINTS

- Safe if used within the recommended doses
- Requires patient cooperation.

INDICATIONS

Any situation where safe operating conditions and adequate analgesia can be provided.

CONTRAINDICATIONS

1. Large or numerous wounds where safe dose is likely to be exceeded
2. Deep wounds requiring exploration and repair of deeper structures
3. Allergy to amide anaesthetics
4. Refusal or poor cooperation, e.g. children
5. Complete heart block
6. Porphyria
7. Infection at injection site – relative contraindication.

PRECAUTIONS

1. Local anaesthesia solutions containing adrenaline may be of occasional use in A&E. They allow an increase in safe dose and decrease immediate bleeding
2. Adrenaline is NOT to be used for hands, feet, ears, nose or penis injuries
3. Allow time for anaesthesia to work, usually 5–10 minutes.

ADVICE TO PATIENTS

Infiltration of local anaesthesia causes transient pain and

discomfort. This can be decreased by slow injection of local anaesthetic which is at room temperature.

METHODS OF LOCAL ANAESTHESIA

1. Local infiltration
   - 1.0% lignocaine commonly used
   - assess for safe dose. For lignocaine 3 mg/kg. A 1.0% solution contains 10 mg/ml, i.e a 70 kg person can have a maximum of 21 ml of 1% lignocaine
   - ensure no allergy to local anaesthesia
   - insert needle to side of wound and ensure no intravascular puncture
   - infiltrate around the wound
   - allow 5–10 minutes for anaesthesia to work
   - use of 0.5% solution or dilution to 0.5% allows larger volumes to be given if required
2. Ring blocks for fingers and toes
   - always use PLAIN lignocaine
   - use 1.0% or 2.0% solution of lignocaine
   - puncture skin to one side of proximal phalanx at level of web
   - advance needle to palmar surface but do not puncture palmar skin
   - ensure no intravascular puncture
   - as needle is withdrawn inject 2 ml
   - repeat on other side of finger
   - allow 5–10 minutes for anaesthesia to work
   - if wound is on dorsum of finger, a further 1 ml can be injected transversely across dorsum of base of finger.

(There are other local anaesthetic techniques, but they are beyond the scope of this book.)

Sutures

KEY POINTS

- Thorough cleaning of wound is essential
- If in doubt, leave wound open.

PREPARATION

1. Ensure adequate light
2. Ensure adequate anaesthesia
3. Ensure help if required.

METHOD

1. Wound cleaning
2. Select appropriate suture material and size
3. Anaesthesia as appropriate
4. Close wound by interrupted suture, making sure that the edges are accurately apposed and everted.

ALTERNATIVES

1. If the wound is deep, the deeper layers may be closed with absorbable sutures
2. When the initial 'bite' of skin is deep, mattress sutures may be used to allow for better opposition.

Choice of suture material

NYLON

The most commonly used suture material for skin in A&E, e.g. Ethilon, Novofil.

Advantages
1. Less tissue reaction
2. Associated with reduced rates of infection
3. Non-absorbable.

Disadvantages
Tendency for knots to slip so a third throw is essential.

SIZES

1. Face 5/0 or 6/0
2. Scalp 3/0
3. Hands 4/0
4. Feet 4/0
5. Legs 3/0
6. Trunk 3/0.

ALTERNATIVES

1. Polypropylene has similar properties to nylon but does not handle as easily
2. Silk handles easily but causes greater tissue reaction and scarring – not for use on the face, but may be acceptable for scalp wounds
3. Absorbable sutures are used for deeper layers:
   - biological materials, e.g. catgut
   - synthetic materials, e.g. Vicryl, Dexon, PDS.

Post suture care and advice

IMMEDIATE CARE

1. Light non-adherent dressing, or leave open
2. Elevation of injured extremity
3. Immobilization and splintage if wound is over a joint, especially extensor surface. However, the advantage of immobilization of the wound must be balanced with the potential for joint stiffness. In general, joint mobilization should start within 24 hours. Any immobilization must be in the position of function.

ADVICE TO PATIENTS

1. Observe for signs of infection:
   - redness
   - increasing pain
   - swelling
   - pyrexia
   - red streaks spreading up extremity (lymphangitis)
2. Review
   - if signs of infection, as above
   - 48–72 hours for high risk wounds
3. Food handlers must be aware of regulations regarding their work and the special dressings required.

REMOVAL OF SUTURES

1. Face 3–5 days
2. Scalp 7–10 days
3. Trunk 10–14 days
4. Arms and legs 10–14 days
5. Hands 7–10 days
6. Over joints 14–21 days.

Steristrips

KEY POINT

- Not always an easy alternative to sutures.

INDICATIONS

1. Small wounds, especially on faces
2. Wounds where skin is too weak to take sutures, e.g. pretibial lacerations.

USEFUL IN

1. Children
2. Flap lacerations
3. Finger injuries
4. Adjunct to sutures, or when sutures removed.

ADVANTAGES

1. Quick
2. Less painful to apply.

DISADVANTAGES

1. Not useful over joints, especially extensor surfaces
2. May peel off, especially if become wet.

METHOD

1. Wound assessment and cleaning
2. Dry surrounding area
3. Need haemostasis to apply Steristrips

4. Tinc. Benz. Co. can be applied to skin to help adhesion, but avoid direct application to wound
5. Place strips at right angles across wound – without tension
6. Glue can be applied to ends of Steristrips to stop them peeling off prematurely.

Tissue adhesive – histoacryl

KEY POINTS

- Accurately approximate epidermis before applying glue
- Do not let glue go on non-skin structures
- Glue only sticks epidermis.

CONTRAINDICATIONS

1. Over joints
2. Deep wounds (leaves dead space for haematoma formation)
3. Close to the eye
4. Moist surfaces, e.g. mucosa
5. Wet surfaces, e.g. bleeding wounds
6. Gaping wounds (dermis is the strength layer and needs to be opposed)
7. Restless or uncooperative patient.

ADVANTAGES

1. Local anaesthetic not required
2. Painless
3. Do not need follow-up for removal
4. Quicker than suturing
5. Does not affect microcirculation, therefore useful for thin flaps.

METHOD OF USE

1. Thoroughly clean the wound
2. Explore wound to ensure no damage to deep structures
3. Local anaesthetic is not required; stinging is usually due to failure to approximate the wound
4. Approximate the wound edges (by simple digital pressure;

in scalp, twists of hair can be pulled across the wound to close it)
5. Drop histoacryl on to approximated wound
6. Apply as spot welds (this leaves gaps in case of haematoma formation or infection)
7. Hold in position for 30–60 seconds.

PRECAUTIONS

1. Always wear gloves – for infection protection and in case you glue yourself to patient
2. Vial of glue can be reused providing it has not touched the patient or been contaminated
3. Do not use in combination with sutures – you will not be able to remove them.

OTHER USES

1. Gluing end of Steristrips (in awkward areas, or to stop children picking ends)
2. Fixing a split nail.

ADVICE TO PATIENTS

1. They can wash the area but must dab it dry, not brush it
2. Do not pick the scab of glue
3. Glue comes off on its own
4. If wound should come apart then return (this usually means that suturing is required)
5. If wound becomes red, painful or any discharge develops, seek medical advice.

Prophylactic antibiotic in wound care

KEY POINTS

- Not used as routine
- Not a substitute for proper wound cleaning.

DEFINITE INDICATIONS

1. Compound fractures
2. Most human and animal bites (see p. 112)
3. Puncture wounds
4. Patients with valvular heart disease or prosthetic valves
5. As part of tetanus prophylaxis in high risk situations (see Antitetanus prophylaxis, p. 106).

RELATIVE INDICATIONS

1. Wounds with marked soiling
2. Late presentation (over six hours)
3. Necrotic tissue.

RECOMMENDED ANTIBIOTICS

1. Flucloxacillin – most widely used
2. Erythromycin – if allergic to penicillin
3. Co-amoxiclav – if high risk of anaerobic involvement, e.g. human bites.

Wound infection

- Prevention is better than cure, so take care in initial wound assessment and cleaning
- May be primary presentation
- Consider retained foreign body.

ASSESSMENT

1. Examine wound and surrounding area for:
   - cellulitis
   - abscess
   - lymphangitis
2. Examine regional lymph nodes
3. Check temperature.

TREATMENT

1. Removal of sutures if present
2. Swab for bacterial culture
3. Thorough cleaning
4. Antiseptic dressing
5. Elevation
6. Antibiotics for cellulitis, lymphangitis or systemic symptoms when no localized collection to drain – usually flucloxacillin
7. Can usually be treated as an outpatient
8. Review in two to three days (cellulitis can be reassessed by marking the initial extent on the skin with an indelible marker).

INDICATION FOR REFERRAL

1. Systemic features of infection

2. Lymph node involvement
3. Severe local symptoms
4. Failure of outpatient treatment.

Foreign bodies in wounds

KEY POINTS

- Can be very difficult to remove
- Be aware of your limitations.

ASSESSMENT

1. History
   - shattered glass
   - high speed metal fragments
   - wound not healing, suspect foreign body
   - patient convinced of possibility of foreign body
   - always listen to the patient
2. Examination
   - direct vision
   - tenderness on palpation of wound
3. Investigations
   - X-rays will detect metal and 99% glass, depending on interface with fluid or air
   - X-rays may detect plastics, stones, grit
   - X-rays will not detect wood

(**NB** Mark site of skin wound with radio-opaque object, e.g. paper clip)
   - ultrasound may be useful for locating some foreign bodies.

MANAGEMENT

1. If easily visible or palpable it can be removed in A&E
   - ensure good light and adequate anaesthesia
   - ideally there should be a bloodless field e.g. a finger tourniquet
   - document removal and show object to patient

- if the particle is wooden, assess for fragmentation
- wash out wound after removal

2. If foreign body cannot be seen or felt,
   - assess degree of difficulty of removal
   - determine whether admission or referral would be better option
3. Tetanus prophylaxis as appropriate
4. If in doubt refer for specialist opinion.

INDICATIONS FOR FURTHER ASSESSMENT

1. Poor cooperation, e.g. child
2. Foreign body near or potentially near vital structures
3. Large foreign bodies
4. Inability to find or remove.

REFERENCE

Wardrope, J. (1996). Foreign bodies in wounds – risk management. *Clinical Risk*, **2**(1), 15–16.

Specific foreign bodies

PROTRUDING PINS/NAILS/SCREWS ETC.

1. Assess deeper structures
2. X-ray to confirm
   - depth
   - bony involvement
   - shape of foreign body
3. Smooth objects may be pulled out gently
4. Screws and irregular objects may need to be dissected out.

FISH HOOKS

1. Local anaesthesia as appropriate
2. Removal
   - push hook through and cut off barb, then pull out smooth remains, or
   - dissect down to barb and withdraw hook intact.

SPLINTER UNDER NAIL

1. It may be possible to use splinter forceps and pull splinter out
2. If unable to grasp the splinter with forceps or if it disintegrates
   - the nail may need to be removed to access the splinter
   - a V-shaped cut in the nail over the splinter
   - a window cut in the nail, which can then be glued back in place after splinter removal.

NB All of the above will require tetanus immunization as appropriate and wound cleaning.

Abrasions

- Superficial skin injury, often very painful.

MANAGEMENT

1. Thorough cleaning is essential (retained dirt leads to tattooing)
2. Remove pieces of grit etc.
3. May need local anaesthetic to allow required cleaning
4. Tetanus immunization as appropriate
5. Non-adherent dressing, e.g. paraffin impregnated gauze.

ALTERNATIVES

1. Facial abrasions can be left exposed after cleaning
2. A dab of povidone iodine may be applied acting both as an antiseptic and a drying agent.

Minor burns

May be treated as outpatients, but first exclude the following:
- burns involving over 15% of body surface area (BSA) in adults
- burns involving over 10% of BSA in children
- full thickness burns involving over 5% of BSA
- significant inhalational injury
- burns involving the airway
- significant intercurrent illness
- burns involving special sites, e.g. perineum, eyes, mouth.

ASSESSMENT

1. History of the event including
   - burning agent
   - time elapsed
   - associated injuries, etc.
2. Examination
   - site
   - size (size can be estimated by using Lund and Browder chart or 'Rule of 9's')
   - depth of burn wound
3. Investigations
   - none needed for uncomplicated burns
   - X-ray for associated injuries as appropriate
   - bacteriology swab for older burns.

TREATMENT

1. Remove burning agent
2. Cold water soaked pads or irrigation
3. Pain relief as required

4. Deroof tense blisters or blisters over joints using sterile needle
5. Dress using paraffin impregnated gauze or non-adherent dressing, e.g. Granuflex
6. Tetanus immunization as appropriate.

ALTERNATIVES

1. Flamazine cream
2. Leave exposed if in area that can be kept clean and dry, e.g. the face.

Burns to special areas

EYES

1. Assess visual acuity
2. Fluorescein to check for corneal abrasions
3. Superficial burns can be treated with chloramphenicol ointment, mydriatic drops and an eye patch
4. Refer for follow-up to an ophthalmology department
5. Chemical burns should be irrigated with at least one litre of saline (best done via an intravenous giving set)
6. More severe burns and all chemical burns, especially alkalis, should be referred immediately.

HANDS

1. Small areas can be treated as for burns in general
2. Larger areas of erythema or burns of uncertain depth can be treated in a Flamazine bag
3. Advise patient that their hand will look macerated on removal of the bag
4. Advise patients to exercise hand to full range of movement and keep hand at shoulder level
5. Reassess after two to three days, when the extent of the burn should be clearer
6. Deroof blisters and dress with paraffin impregnated gauze, keeping the fingers separate.

FACE

1. Assess severity, taking particular care of the airway and eyes
2. Swelling may be dramatic – warn the patient. If leads to (or may lead to) difficulty in eating, talking or swallowing, will need admission
3. Severe burns should be referred for admission

4. Minor burns are treated by cleaning and exposure. They can be dabbed with povidone iodine
5. Flamazine cream should not be applied because of skin staining
6. Vaseline/white soft paraffin may be used as an alternative.

Specific minor burns

Sunburn

KEY POINTS

- Often widespread but usually limited to erythema
- There may be some blistering.

ASSESSMENT AND TREATMENT

Treat as for any other burn.

ADVICE

Use this opportunity to advise on sun screen, wearing head protection and protective clothes etc.

Electrical burns

KEY POINTS

- Extent and damage will depend on voltage of supply
- Domestic supply is low voltage
- Burn is usually full thickness
- Consider effects of electric shock.

ASSESSMENT

1. Examine for associated injuries
2. Check for proximal muscle tenderness
3. Check nerve function in the limb
4. Examine burn wound, but bear in mind that tissue damage may be below the surface and may worsen over the first few days.

TREATMENT

1. Consider urgent referral for excision and grafting
2. In the meantime, dressing and tetanus immunization as for other burns.

NB Because of the high risk of complications with high voltage burns, all should be referred.

Chemical burns

KEY POINTS

- Many agents continue to burn
- Seek Poison Centre advice if required.

MANAGEMENT

1. Copious irrigation with cold water.
2. Do not neutralize chemicals, as the ensuing reaction will often cause further burning
3. In general, treat thereafter as for any burn.

SPECIFIC CHEMICALS

1. Glues and adhesives can generally be left to peel off spontaneously as they do not damage the skin
2. Adherent bitumen should be left in place, but ensure that it has cooled down completely
3. Hydrofluoric acid – lavage followed by topical calcium gluconate gel
4. Phenol – consider referral if the area is large because of absorption and risk of renal damage. Copious water is better than delaying to find some glycol irrigant
5. Phosphorous burns – either keep immersed or under continuous spray. Refer to specialist centre for advice
6. Cement is highly caustic and adheres to the skin. Irrigate thoroughly and scrub the area if required. Ensure all cement is removed.

Facial wounds

- Because of rich blood supply can be sutured up to 24 hours after injury
- Consider cosmetic implications.

ASSESSMENT

1. Check underlying nerves
   - facial nerve – muscles of facial expressions
   - trigeminal nerve – sensory to face
2. Muscles of mastication
3. For wounds around the eye, test for:
   - visual acuity
   - ocular integrity
4. Examine for underlying bony injury
5. Remember salivary glands and parotid duct.

MANAGEMENT

1. Adequate anaesthesia
2. Thorough cleaning including scrubbing to remove dirt which may lead to tattooing
3. Close deep wounds in layers:
   - deep 4/0–5/0 absorbable
   - skin 5/0–6/0 monofilament non-absorbable, e.g. nylon
   - Steristrips.

CAUTION

1. Ensure that the following structures are lined up carefully:
   - hair-line
   - eyebrows
   - nasolabial folds

- nostril rims
- columella
- philtrum
- vermilion borders

2. If first attempt is not satisfactory, remove sutures and try again
3. Wetting the lip makes the vermilion borders easier to see.

ADVICE TO PATIENTS

1. Dressings are not usually needed (sticking plasters may be used for children)
2. Keep the wound clean
3. Final result of treatment may not be evaluated for at least six months, when the scar has 'settled'
4. Once stitches removed, massage of wound with bland cream may help cosmetic appearance.

INDICATIONS FOR REFERRAL

1. When lack of patient cooperation hinders a good cosmetic result, e.g. children
2. Damage to underlying structures
3. Wounds involving
   - margins of eyelids
   - angle of mouth
   - significant skin loss.

Pretibial lacerations

- Often following a trivial injury
- Common in elderly people where pretibial skin is very thin
- When a flap laceration is present the apex may have a compromised blood supply, especially if the flap is distally based
- Healing is often very slow.

ASSESSMENT

1. Size and depth of wound
2. Viability of flap
3. Underlying bony injury
4. General condition of patients, e.g.
   - dependent oedema
   - peripheral vascular status
   - varicose veins
5. Check patient's regular medications, especially steroid usage.

MANAGEMENT

1. Clean wound
2. Bring edges of wound as close as possible without any tension
3. Use Steristrips or glue, not sutures
4. Cover residual open areas with paraffin impregnated gauze (but this must not be laid over Steristrips)
5. Tetanus immunization as appropriate
6. Advise patient on keeping leg elevated but stress importance of calf exercises
7. Graduated compression stockings may be useful if leg is swollen for any reason.

FOLLOW-UP

1. Review after three to four days, according to local practice
2. Avoid removing steristrips until at least 10 days
3. Warn that healing often takes several weeks
4. If healing is delayed or skin defect is large, consider referral for grafting.

Puncture wounds

KEY POINTS

- Especially common in hands and feet, e.g. 'trod on a nail'
- Remember what the puncturing object has passed through, e.g. shoes, socks etc.

ASSESSMENT

1. Accurate history
2. Examination of the skin wound (often unremarkable)
3. Examine for injury to deeper structures.

MANAGEMENT

1. Clean surrounding area and soak site with antiseptic
2. Irrigation of wound with sterile saline using a needle and syringe
3. Tetanus immunization as appropriate
4. Prophylactic antibiotics
5. Advise patient of signs of infection, and to return if these develop.

ALTERNATIVES

'Coning' of wound using size 11 blade under local anaesthetic.

INDICATION FOR FURTHER ASSESSMENT

1. Damage to underlying structure
2. Restriction of joint movement (suggesting capsular penetration)
3. Established infection.

Section 2
Minor trauma

Acute neck sprain

KEY POINTS

- May occur spontaneously ('wry neck', 'torticollis')
- Pain and stiffness are maximal 24–48 hours after injury
- If road traffic accident at >30 miles per hour, fall >10 feet, injury above the clavicles, assume cervical spine injury and immobilize with hard collar, sand bags and tape.

ASSESSMENT

1. Traumatic:
   - ask about mechanism of injury, onset and radiation of pain, any associated symptoms
   - full neurological examination
   - palpate for tenderness while head and neck are manually immobilized by an assistant
   - cervical spine X-rays if any neurological abnormality, bony/midline tenderness or mechanism criteria as above.
2. Non-traumatic:
   - ask about onset and duration of pain, associated symptoms including sore throat, dysphagia, neck swelling, temperature, swallowed foreign bodies
   - examine neck for tenderness, swelling, nodes
   - assess range of movement of neck and shoulders
   - examine ENT, assess swallowing, check temperature
   - full neurological examination
   - cervical spine X-rays as indicated for trauma
   - soft tissue neck X-ray for swallowed foreign bodies (see p. 139), retropharyngeal swelling.

INDICATORS OF NEED FOR FURTHER INVESTIGATION/ASSESSMENT

1. Abnormalities on cervical spine X-ray; keep immobilized and seek further opinion
2. Evidence of retropharyngeal infection; refer to ENT
3. Retained foreign body (p. 139).

MANAGEMENT

1. Treat specific causes identified during assessment
2. If X-rays normal, give nonsteroidal anti-inflammatory drug and advice on neck exercises to prevent further stiffening
3. Early physiotherapy for traumatic causes may help prevent later problems
4. Support neck with pillow or rolled up towel at night
5. Stress importance of good posture (hold the chin back).

ALTERNATIVES

Other acceptable forms of management include soft collars, which are of no proven benefit but some patients find them comforting.

Acute tenosynovitis

Most frequently affects tendons and sheaths around the wrist joint but can present at any site.

ASSESSMENT

1. The pain may be described as grating or crunching if crepitus is present, or sharp if not. It is aggravated by particular movements according to the tendon affected
2. Look for erythema, swelling and tenderness along the line of the tendon. Crepitus may be felt on movement
3. Assess for other injuries
4. Check temperature and look for signs of infection.

INDICATORS OF NEED FOR FURTHER INVESTIGATION/ASSESSMENT

If doubt about the possibility of soft tissue infection exists, treat simultaneously with antibiotics and arrange review in 24–48 hours.

MANAGEMENT

1. X-rays may be required if bony tenderness is prominent
2. Nonsteroidal anti-inflammatory drugs, topical or oral, provide the most effective relief, provided they are not contraindicated
3. A short period of rest and support may be required, e.g. tubigrip, sling, depending on site. Symptoms usually settle in 48 hours.

ALTERNATIVES

Other acceptable forms of management include:
1. In severe cases, a period of immobilization in a splint or plaster for one to two weeks may be required
2. Local corticosteroid injection can settle inflammation but is usually reserved for severe cases.

Ankle injuries

- Frequent cause of attendance at A&E departments
- Majority settle quickly with appropriate treatment
- Injury to other structures around the ankle will be missed unless examined for specifically
- Fracture dislocations at the ankle with impaired circulation (loss of foot pulses or blanching of the skin over pressure points) need to be reduced as soon as possible, usually prior to X-ray, to restore circulation and ensure tissue viability.

ASSESSMENT

1. Ask about the mechanism of injury. The most frequent mechanism is inversion causing injury to the talofibular ligament
2. Is the patient able to weight bear now and could they do so immediately after injury?
3. Examine the ankle, looking particularly at the site of any swelling, bruising or tenderness
4. Examine the calcaneum (injured in falls from height), specific calcaneal views should be requested on X-ray if damage is suspected
5. Examine the Achilles tendon, feeling for gaps in the tendon above the heel. Assess passive and active plantarflexion of the foot
6. Examine the foot, particularly the fifth metatarsal which may be fractured in an inversion injury
7. Assess distal neurovascular function.

INDICATORS OF NEED FOR FURTHER INVESTIGATION/ASSESSMENT

X rays will be required if:

1. The patient has been unable to weightbear from the time of injury or can walk less than five steps now
2. There is bony tenderness
3. There is marked swelling or bruising
4. There is deformity or marked restriction of movement.

Patients with fractures should be referred according to local policy. In general, avulsion fractures of the tip of the malleoli can be treated as sprains (see below).

Complete or partial rupture of the Achilles tendon should be referred to the orthopaedic team for management.

MANAGEMENT

1. Fracture dislocation with impaired circulation:
   - provide analgesia such as entonox or intravenous opiates
   - apply traction to the foot to restore the foot and ankle to a neutral position
   - recheck circulation
   - apply a below-knee splint or backslab
   - arrange X-ray and referral to orthopaedic team.
2. X-rays normal:
   - apply a support bandage to the affected ankle
   - give simple analgesics and advice on rest, ice and elevation (see soft tissue injuries)
   - a walking stick or crutches may be required for a short period (e.g. two to seven days).

ALTERNATIVES

Other acceptable forms of management include:

1. Patients with severe sprains may benefit from a period of immobilization in a below-knee plaster cast. Appropriate follow-up should be arranged
2. Early physiotherapy can help to restore normal gait and proprioception.

Bruised chest and fractured ribs

KEY POINTS

- Only need X-ray if suspect a complication
- Pain relief is vital and must be adequate
- Breathing exercises and no smoking prevent chest infection.

ASSESSMENT

1. Check for evidence of intrathoracic injury
2. Check for respiratory compromise
3. Exclude other injuries, especially intra-abdominal injury in fractures of lower ribs.

INDICATORS OF NEED FOR CHEST X-RAY

1. High energy accident
2. Localized tenderness over the sternum
3. Suspicion of pneumothorax, haemothorax, flail chest
4. Pre-existing severe respiratory disease
5. Injury to upper three ribs or clavicle.

INDICATIONS FOR ADMISSION

1. Complication
2. Inadequate pain control
3. Unable to exclude intra-abdominal injury
4. Multiple rib fractures or fractures of ribs 1–3.

MANAGEMENT

Providing complications have been excluded:
1. Strong analgesia, e.g. dihydrocodeine

2. Breathing exercises every four hours. As deep a breath as possible, hold for two seconds then breath out fully and repeat ten times. Best done 30–45 minutes after taking analgesia
3. No strapping.

AFTERCARE

1. Minimize smoking
2. Continue exercises until pain-free
3. If need to cough or sneeze press open hand firmly against injured area to minimize pain
4. Advise severe pain often persists for one to two weeks, and some pain for four to eight weeks
5. If cough up blood should go to A&E immediately; if cough up discoloured sputum should contact GP.

Child not using upper limb

KEY POINTS

- Usually in a child less than five years old
- Often no witnessed injury and may be delayed presentation (consider NAI)
- Child noted to be holding affected arm by side or favouring other arm
- Most commonly pulled elbow or greenstick fracture clavicle or radius.

ASSESSMENT

1. History of pulling injury suggests pulled elbow (p. 83)
2. Ask about duration of symptoms, localize pain if possible
3. Inspect whole arm, clavicle to hand, for abnormalities
4. Assess active and passive movements of the limb
5. Assess neurovascular function
6. If no history of injury check temperature and skin for signs of infection and nodes. Consider other illnesses, e.g. sickle cell disease.

INDICATORS OF NEED FOR FURTHER INVESTIGATION/ASSESSMENT

1. Consider NAI (p. 76)
2. Febrile or septic child will need to be admitted.

MANAGEMENT

1. Pulled elbow (p. 83)
2. Most cases will require X-ray. It is often impossible to localize the site of injury in a young child and X-rays of the whole limb may be required
3. If X-rays are normal and the child well, discharge home

with simple analgesia. Child should return in 24 hours if still not using the limb normally (earlier if worse or unwell).

Closed soft tissue injuries

KEY POINTS

- May cause prolonged morbidity
- Presentation often delayed – 'I thought it would get better'.

ASSESSMENT

1. Most common symptoms are pain, swelling and loss of function
2. Ask about mechanism of injury, previous injury/illness affecting site
3. Look for distribution of swelling and bruise, note any deformity
4. Locate the area of maximum tenderness
5. Assess range of movement for limitation due to pain, or excessive mobility due to ligament rupture
6. Assess distal nurovascular function
7. X-ray if fracture not excluded clinically.

INDICATORS OF NEED FOR FURTHER INVESTIGATION/ASSESSMENT

1. Excess mobility indicating fracture or ruptured ligament
2. Fractures
3. Evidence of loss of sensation or circulation.

MANAGEMENT

R.I.C.E.
1. Rest. An initial period of rest for 24–48 hours. During this time gentle non-weightbearing, non-resisted exercise should be started
2. Ice. Applied to the affected area for roughly 10 minutes

each hour for the first day. Apply as either ice cubes or bag of frozen peas wrapped in a towel
3. Compression. Support bandages may help to reduce swelling and provide some support. The effects are however shortlived. Beware causing excess compression over flexed joints
4. Elevation. The most effective way of reducing swelling
5. Return to normal activities gradually, guided by pain/discomfort
6. Physiotherapy is particularly useful for some injuries
7. Nonsteroidal anti-inflammatory drugs provide pain relief. If contraindicated, paracetamol or paracetamol/codeine mixtures can be used.

Domestic violence

- Detection of domestic violence is an important aspect of preventative emergency medicine
- Most victims are women but it affects all classes, races and religions
- Presentation can take many forms.

ASSESSMENT

1. It may present as injury, attempted suicide, depression, overdose, abdominal pain, gynaecological problems or multiple minor complaints
2. Be suspicious if partner answers all the questions
3. Presentation may be delayed and history may be vague or reluctantly given
4. Interviewing in private and asking directly about domestic violence is important
5. Record all injuries carefully
6. Find out if others, e.g. children, are at risk.

MANAGEMENT

1. Treat medical condition as required
2. Offer to contact friends or relatives
3. Offer assistance in finding place of safety, e.g. refuge
4. Call duty social worker
5. Enquire whether patient wants police involved – advise if there is a specialist domestic violence unit
6. If wishes to go home, give written advice on who to contact
7. Inform general practitioner of circumstances
8. Give contact numbers of local and national helplines (e.g. Women's Aid, 0117 963 3542).

All the above can be usefully combined in an information leaflet.

Ear injuries

Major goal is protection of cartilage.

ASSESSMENT

1. Examine pinna
2. Beware in assessing bleeding from the ear. Remember – head injury and basal skull fracture
3. Perforation of the ear drum
4. Local wound in auditory canal.

MANAGEMENT

1. Thorough cleaning
2. Tetanus immunization as appropriate
3. Local anaesthesia can be provided by a field block around the entire base of the ear.

Simple laceration (not involving the cartilage) – may be sutured using 5/0 monofilament nonabsorbable sutures.

Skin loss or *cartilage involvement* – refer for further treatment.

Subperichondrial haematoma

1. Will lead to cauliflower ear if left untreated
2. Attempt aspiration under aseptic conditions using 18 gauge needle
3. Apply pressure with padding behind the ear and cotton wool formed to shape of convolutions of pinna
4. Risk of recurrence is high so early referral is needed.

Split ear lobe

1. If the edges are fresh – suture
2. If the edges are epithelialized, they will need to be reopened prior to suturing (this is not an emergency procedure).

Fingertip injuries

KEY POINTS

- Refers to injuries of distal phalanx beyond insertion of tendons
- Usually caused by crush injury
- Aim to provide good function.

ASSESSMENT

1. Examine nail and nail bed
2. Skin of pulp and tip
3. Viability of tissue
4. Confirm distal interphalangeal joint is not involved
5. Most will require an X-ray to assess any bony involvement.

MANAGEMENT

1. Thorough cleaning
2. Local anaesthesia, e.g. ring block to allow treatment and as a method of pain relief
3. Surgical repair may need a tourniquet, e.g. thin rubber catheter or finger of surgeons' gloves rolled down to base of finger
4. Elevate
5. Analgesia
6. Exercise whole hand
7. Desensitization (tapping the end of the finger to prevent hypersensitivity).

OPTIONS

Children may be treated conservatively with cleaning and dressing. The fingertip regrows and the result is good.

Simple skin loss (no bone or nail bed involvement):
1. Dress using paraffin impregnated gauze
2. Alternatives are Flamazine dressing, Granuflex™.

'Burst' lacerations

1. Should be approximated using Steristrips, if possible
2. Suturing may lead to an increase in tension
3. Elevate in high arm sling.

Nail bed injuries

1. The nail should be removed and any laceration sutured using 4/0–5/0 absorbable suture
2. The nail should be cleaned, replaced and secured with Steristrips
3. If the nail is lost or damaged, the sterile foil from the suture packet may be used as a dressing.

Partial amputation (with bone exposed)

1. The bone will need to be covered
2. Refer for specialist management, e.g. various grafting or finger-shortening procedures.

INDICATORS OF NEED FOR FURTHER INVESTIGATION AND ADMISSION

1. Exposed bone
2. Exposed tendon
3. Occupations requiring very fine sensation in tip.

Fractured nose

- X-rays do not alter management
- Septal haematomas must be recognized and treated early.

ASSESSMENT

1. Check patency of nostrils and inspect for septal haematomas which appear as red swellings on the nasal septum
2. Assess for other injuries, especially to the rest of the face and eyes.

INDICATORS OF NEED FOR FURTHER INVESTIGATION/ASSESSMENT

1. Septal haematomas require immediate drainage to prevent late complications
2. Evidence of bony injury extending further onto the face will require more detailed assessment.

MANAGEMENT

1. Epistaxis can usually be stopped by pinching the fleshy portion of the nose firmly for ten minutes
2. X-rays are not required. If the nose appears fractured clinically, make arrangements according to local policy for the patient to be reviewed in five to seven days time. Most of the swelling will then have settled and an assessment of the need for surgery can be made
3. Provide analgesia and tetanus prophylaxis as required.

Fractured sternum

KEY POINTS

- Can be associated with serious intrathoracic pathology
- Some cases can be safely managed at home
- All cases need X-ray assessment and ECG.

ASSESSMENT

1. Ask about mechanism of injury
2. Check for injuries elsewhere
3. Assess degree of respiratory compromise before and after analgesia
4. Tenderness should be well localized; if not look for other injuries
5. Check for evidence of other chest injuries
6. Ask about pre-existing respiratory or cardiovascular disease.

MANAGEMENT

1. Strong analgesia, e.g. dihydrocodeine
2. Breathing exercises every four hours. As deep a breath as possible, hold for two seconds then breath out fully; repeat ten times. Best done 30–45 minutes after taking analgesia. This may be made less uncomfortable by hugging a pillow firmly against the chest whilst undertaking the exercises.

INDICATORS OF NEED FOR FURTHER INVESTIGATION AND ADMISSION

1. High energy mechanism of injury
2. Abnormal ECG
3. Abnormal chest X-ray (in addition to the fracture)
4. Inadequate pain relief
5. Continuing respiratory distress after analgesia
6. Pre-existing respiratory disease.

Fractured toes

- Can usually be managed without X-ray
- Need to differentiate from dislocated toe.

ASSESSMENT

1. Look for deformity, including rotation
2. Check circulation and sensation
3. Check tendon function
4. If no movement in a joint, suspect dislocation
5. Assess any wounds
6. X-ray if possibility of dislocation, gross swelling or deformity.

INDICATORS OF NEED FOR FURTHER INVESTIGATION AND ASSESSMENT/REFERRAL

1. Deformity not corrected
2. Unstable fracture
3. Tendon injury
4. Gross open fracture.

MANAGEMENT

1. If deformed, rotated or dislocated, reduce under digital nerve block
2. Trephine any subungual haematoma
3. Clean any wounds
4. Give flucloxacillin for five days, if compound fracture
5. Analgesia
6. Neighbour strapping
7. Elevate foot as much as possible, avoid standing still or sitting with foot dependent

8. Encourage normal gait
9. Elevate foot whenever seated
10. Keep strapping in place for two weeks or until pain-free, whichever is earlier
11. Fracture clinic only for compound, displaced or great toe fractures
12. Seek medical advice if pain worsens or more than an ache in two weeks.

Fractures

KEY POINTS

- The main symptom is pain, which can be relieved by immobilization of the fracture and analgesics
- Symptoms and signs may be more subtle in children
- Pain from one injury may mask another.

ASSESSMENT

1. Examine the bone affected and the joints above and below
2. Look for swelling, bruising, deformity. Assess for mobility which may be limited or excessive
3. Look for wounds
4. Assess distal neurovascular function
5. Have a lower threshold for X-ray in children – greenstick fractures often have subtle signs.

INDICATORS OF NEED FOR FURTHER INVESTIGATION/ASSESSMENT

1. Gross deformity
2. Involvement of joint surfaces
3. Reduced sensation or circulation distal to the fracture
4. Compound fractures
5. Epiphyseal injuries.

MANAGEMENT

1. Provide analgesia (e.g. entonox, oral or intravenous analgesics as appropriate)
2. Reduce immediately if there is neurovascular compromise
3. Immobilize the limb in a sling or splint. Very mobile fractures are best immobilized in plaster of Paris backslab or splint prior to X-ray

4. Compound wounds require covering with a sterile dressing, tetanus prophylaxis if indicated (see p. 106), antibiotic cover
5. Arrange X-ray
6. Treatment depends on individual fracture type.

High pressure injection injuries

KEY POINTS

- Wound does not reflect severity
- Needs urgent exploration/decompression.

Can be caused by high pressure air lines, paint guns, moulding injectors, hydraulic lines, grease guns, diesel fuel jets, compressor lines. The substance injected may be air, grease, hydraulic fluid, paint, solvents, oil.

ASSESSMENT

1. Pain initially is poor indicator of severity
2. Entry wound may be small, check for contamination
3. Check tension in surrounding tissues
4. Check for palpable material spreading from wound, e.g. surgical emphysema
5. Check circulation and sensation distally
6. Check for specific problems of substance injected – contact manufacturers or Poisons Information Service.

INDICATORS OF NEED FOR FURTHER INVESTIGATION/ASSESSMENT

1. X-ray if radio-opaque material injected
2. If neurovascular deficit needs emergency decompression, perform before transfer if possible
3. All cases need referral for urgent exploration, wound toilet and decompression.

MANAGEMENT PENDING EXPLORATION

1. Elevate the limb
2. Analgesia

3. Broad spectrum antibiotics
4. Tetanus cover
5. Do not close wound
6. Do not infiltrate with local anaesthetic as this will increase tissue pressure
7. Contact manufacturers or Poisons Information Service about specific substance injected.

Intraoral lacerations

- Generally heal very well.

ASSESSMENT

1. Note extent and size of wound
2. Examine for associated injuries, e.g. teeth, jaw etc.

MANAGEMENT

1. Tetanus immunization as appropriate
2. Prophylactic antibiotics, e.g. Co-Amoxiclav
3. Mouthwashes and oral hygiene advice
4. Only suture if very large or actively bleeding.

Tongue

1. As for intraoral lacerations
2. Small cuts can be left to heal unaided
3. Large cuts or those involving the edges will need suturing and therefore referral to an oral surgeon.

Gums

1. Can usually be left to heal unaided
2. Attention to any dental injury as appropriate.

'Through and through' lacerations of lip

1. Thorough wound cleaning
2. Skin closure in layers
3. Definite indication for antibiotics
4. Mucosal surface may be left unsutured
5. Mouth washes and oral hygiene advice.

Knee injuries

KEY POINTS

- Always consider hip and spine problems in assessing knee pain
- Swelling may be due to
    blood – often immediate or early in onset
    synovial fluid – more delayed in onset, e.g. overnight
- Early examination in acutely swollen knee is often un-reliable.

ASSESSMENT

1. History
    - mechanism of injury
    - location of pain
    - locking – inability to fully extend the knee
    - giving way
2. Examination
    - tenderness
    - swelling/effusion
    - range of movement
    - specific examination (if possible) for collateral ligaments, cruciate ligaments and menisci
3. Investigations
    - X-ray.

INDICATIONS FOR X-RAY

1. Age over 55 years
2. Tenderness over fibula head
3. Isolated patella tenderness
4. Inability to flex to 90°

5. Inability to weight-bear immediately and time of examination
6. Penetrating injury.

MANAGEMENT

Early swelling
1. This is assumed to be blood until proved otherwise
2. Discuss with orthopaedic team
3. Admit/Fracture Clinic as per local policy
4. Immobilize as per orthopaedic advice.

Delayed swelling
1. A large tense effusion may be aspirated. If blood is aspirated treat as for early swelling
2. A small effusion, or following aspiration of synovial fluid, can be treated conservatively, i.e.
   - rest
   - ice
   - elevation
   - nonsteroidal anti-inflammatories
   - early physiotherapy.
3. Follow-up according to local practice.

Limping child

KEY POINTS

- History of trauma is often unreliable – children often fall, parents often rationalize a limp to a fall
- Think of NAI.

DIFFERENTIAL DIAGNOSIS

1. Acute arthritis
2. Acute osteomyelitis
3. Bone/soft tissue tumour
4. Fracture, especially tibia
5. Irritable hip
6. Leukaemia
7. Perthes' disease
8. Septic arthritis
9. Sickle cell disease
10. Slipped femoral epiphysis.

ASSESSMENT

1. History; trauma, onset, high temperature, other illness
2. Past medical history; previous episodes, family history, had sickle test
3. Inspect for any localized swelling, bruising, deformity
4. Examine the whole leg and pelvis
5. Remember to look for minor complaints of the sole of foot, e.g. verruca, laceration, foreign body
6. Palpate for localized tenderness, warmth
7. Check range of movement of all joints
8. Observe the child whilst playing and trying to walk.

INDICATORS OF NEED FOR FURTHER INVESTIGATION/ASSESSMENT

1. Admit if febrile, toxic, severe muscle spasm
2. Most cases will need X-ray. Unless there is a definite well localized problem, X-ray the whole limb
3. Hip ultrasound is useful to exclude any effusion and to guide aspiration to exclude septic arthritis
4. If cause not apparent on X-ray and child is unwell, then take blood for FBC, ESR, blood culture and sickle screen and admit.

MANAGEMENT OF CASE WITH NORMAL X-RAY, AFEBRILE, SYSTEMICALLY WELL CHILD

1. Ensure no further blood tests required
2. Advise rest
3. Regular paracetamol or ibuprofen
4. Review after 24 hours
5. Return earlier if child becomes febrile, becomes systemically unwell or parents are concerned.

Low grade pyrexia with minimal joint pain and no systemic symptoms, with all other investigations normal, can be managed at home as above. All other cases should be referred for orthopaedic opinion.

Lost teeth

Loss of permanent anterior teeth leads to obvious disfigurement. These teeth are frequently injured in sport, assaults or road traffic accidents.

KEY POINTS

- Replacement of primary (milk) teeth is not required as the risk of aspiration outweighs the benefits of reimplantation
- Replacement is contraindicated in the presence of fracture of the tooth, risk factors for subacute bacterial endocarditis (e.g. rheumatic fever, valvular or septal heart defects), or risk factors for aspiration (e.g. head injury with loss of consciousness).

ASSESSMENT

Check for contraindications to reimplantation as above.

INDICATORS OF NEED FOR FURTHER INVESTIGATION/ASSESSMENT

All patients in whom a tooth is replaced should be seen by a dental practitioner as soon as practicable.

MANAGEMENT

1. First aid advice; the patient should endeavour to replace the tooth immediately and then seek dental care. If they are unable to replace the tooth it should be stored in milk or saliva (in the buccal sulcus)
2. Clean the tooth with normal saline and inspect for fractures
3. Push the tooth firmly into the socket and hold the socket margins around it for one minute

4. Hold the tooth in position with a temporary splint or by the patient biting gently on it, until dental care can be arranged
5. Prescribe penicillin (or erythromycin if allergic)
6. Provide tetanus prophylaxis as required.

Mallet finger

KEY POINTS

- Occurs following a stubbing injury when the extensor tendon is avulsed from the base of the distal phalanx
- The bony attachment of the tendon may be avulsed.

ASSESSMENT

1. Classic mallet deformity – flexion at DIP joint, with no active extension but full range of passive movement
2. No active extension, but is usually pain-free with full passive extension
3. X-ray to check for bony injury.

MANAGEMENT

Maintain distal interphalangeal joint in extension for six weeks using commercially available mallet finger splint.

ADVICE TO PATIENTS

1. Splint must be worn at all times
2. When washing keep extended passively
3. Follow up at Hand Clinic/Fracture Clinic according to local practice
4. Some permanent deformity may remain but rarely causes disability.

INDICATION FOR REFERRAL

Large fragments of bone may need to be surgically reattached.

Muscle haematoma

KEY POINTS

- Carefully check muscle function to exclude rupture
- Soft tissue tumours are rare but often present after minor trauma.

ASSESSMENT

1. Assess for integrity of muscle
2. Enquire about previous injuries
3. Find out about pre-existing symptoms in the area
4. Ask about drugs affecting clotting, e.g. warfarin, aspirin
5. Any evidence of bleeding disorder.

INDICATORS OF NEED FOR FURTHER INVESTIGATION/ASSESSMENT

1. If bony tenderness or pain on stressing bone then undertake X-ray
2. If does not feel typical of haematoma then X-ray and arrange referral for further investigation
3. If muscle function absent, refer to orthopaedic surgeon for repair.

MANAGEMENT

1. Apply cold compress to reduce pain and swelling
2. Ibuprofen
3. Rest and elevate the limb whilst pain severe
   - crutches for lower limb
   - sling for upper limb
4. Gentle exercises to all joints of affected limb every two hours
5. Strapping is controversial. Used immediately may stop

increase in haematoma formation. If prolonged, restricts activity and rarely maintains true compression
6. As pain subsides begin active exercise without resistance, include progressive stretching exercises
7. Refer for physiotherapy/ultrasound.

AFTERCARE

1. Active exercise, avoiding resistance until pain-free
2. Progressive stretching exercises
3. Only return to sport when pain resolved, full muscle length achieved and fully fit
4. Continue stretching exercises prior to sport, indefinitely.

Non-accidental injury

- Know your local policy
- If in doubt refer to paediatrician or social services
- Always be suspicious and then exclude NAI.

SUSPICIOUS FINDINGS

1. History:
   - delay in presentation without adequate explanation
   - change in story with time, or between individuals
   - mechanism of injury not compatible with child's age
   - known history of abuse
   - abnormal parental behaviour, lack of concern
   - frequent injuries or medical attendances
2. Examination:
   - findings not consistent with history
   - injuries of varying ages
   - signs of neglect
   - specific injuries:
     - bites
     - blunt abdominal trauma
     - oral frenulum tear
     - pattern burns
     - pattern/fingermark bruises
     - perineal injuries
     - petechial haemorrhage in upper body
     - retinal haemorrhage
     - subdural haematoma
3. Investigations:
   - skull fracture
   - long bone fracture in child not yet walking
   - multiple injuries of varying age
   - unexplained injuries.

FAMILY RISK FACTORS

Young, unmarried parents, personality disorder, criminal record, social isolation, mental illness, other members of family victims of child abuse.

NB Beware – NAI can and does occur in all socio-economic groups, all ethnic groups and in low risk families.

MANAGEMENT

1. Ensure child and siblings are safe
2. Report to appropriate authority immediately – either social services or paediatrician
3. Document all history taking and clinical findings carefully.

DIFFERENTIAL DIAGNOSIS

1. Osteogenesis imperfecta
2. Idiopathic thrombocytopaenia purpura
3. Leukaemia
4. Other bleeding disorders.

Penis trapped in zip fastener

KEY POINTS

- The patient's confidence is vital
- Release can usually be achieved with adequate local anaesthesia.

MANAGEMENT

1. Anaesthetize the foreskin. This can be achieved with EMLA cream (remember it takes 30–60 minutes to become effective). Alternatively, local anaesthesia can be infiltrated around the base of the penis
2. Reverse the zip
3. Unless bleeding, the skin does not require suturing
4. Daily bath until healed, ensuring foreskin is fully retracted each time
5. Apply white soft paraffin to unhealed area after bathing.

ALTERNATIVES

One
1. Anaesthetize as above
2. Cut the zip between the teeth just above the zipper
3. Advance the zipper so it slides off the cut end.

Two
1. Cut the zip between the teeth just above the zipper
2. Cut along the material of the zip at the base of the teeth
3. Tease the loose teeth out of the zipper – this can be made easier by opening up the slots on the side of the zipper using circlip pliers.

Plaster of Paris: cast advice

KEY POINT

Everyone fitted with a cast must be given advice, verbal and written, on potential complications.

CARE OF POP CAST

1. The POP cast takes 24–48 hours to dry fully. Until that time it must be supported in a sling or on a pillow
2. You should not put weight on a leg plaster until told you can do so
3. Do not get the POP cast wet
4. Do not put anything inside your plaster cast. Do not try to scratch inside with anything.
5. Exercise all joints that are not enclosed in the plaster to stop stiffness and reduce swelling.

WHEN TO RETURN

Sometimes the swelling in the plaster causes problems with the circulation. The risk of this can be decreased by keeping the limb elevated as much as possible in the first 48 hours.

Patient should return immediately if:
1. Fingers/toes go blue
2. Numbness or paraesthesia in distal limb
3. Increasing pain under plaster cast.

Plaster of Paris: pain under cast

KEY POINTS

- Always carefully assess pain under a POP cast
- Worsening pain or pain not relieved by simple analgesia always has a cause
- Assess potential mobility of fracture before removing a cast, e.g. less than 14 days since diagnosis, fracture needing manipulation, comminuted fracture
- If in doubt, elevate the limb, split the cast and refer to team caring for fracture.

ASSESSMENT

1. Ask about elevation and analgesia
2. Check POP for tightness
3. Look for distal oedema
4. Check circulation distally
5. Check sensation distally
6. Remove POP and inspect for signs of compartment syndrome, DVT, friction and infection. If fracture is recent then consider bivalving or window in POP.

COMPARTMENT SYNDROME

1. Symptoms often in excess of signs
2. May be due to constriction of the plaster or from swelling
3. Characterized by pain, pressure, paresis, paraesthesia
4. Think of diagnosis in any pain not relieved by simple analgesics.

TREATMENT

1. Immediately elevate the limb
2. Split the cast and all layers of padding etc. so that skin is visible along whole length of cast
3. If symptoms not relieved within a few minutes, remove plaster completely and consider need for surgical decompression
4. Give analgesia cautiously until decision for surgery.

Post-concussion syndrome

KEY POINTS

- Common after head injury and a cause of much anxiety
- Diagnosis of exclusion
- Be especially cautious with elderly people and alcoholics, in whom there is a greater risk of chronic subdural haematoma.

ASSESSMENT

1. History
   - headache
   - dizziness
   - lethargy
   - lack of concentration

   All of the above can be caused by other post-head injury complications Note the time scale and pattern of symptoms.
2. Examination
   - check vital signs
   - level of consciousness
   - pupillary reactions
   - fundi
   - localizing neurological signs

   All the above will be normal in post-concussion syndrome.

MANAGEMENT

1. If any suspicious clinical features found or 'at risk' patients (e.g. elderly or alcoholics), consider further referral
2. If no abnormal clinical findings
   - reassurance
   - symptomatic treatment, e.g. analgesia
   - psychotherapy (if major interference with work etc.).

Pulled elbow

KEY POINTS

- Occurs in children under five years of age
- Caused by traction of fully extended elbow, e.g. lifting or swinging child by wrists
- See also 'Child not using upper limb' (p. 48).

ASSESSMENT

1. Child refuses to use or move arm
2. Holds forearm in pronation
3. Only tenderness is over area of radial head
4. Always consider whether it could be a supracondylar fracture.

INDICATORS OF NEED FOR X-RAY BEFORE REDUCTION

1. Atypical history
2. Bony tenderness
3. Swelling, bruising around elbow.

MANAGEMENT

1. Tell parents what you are going to do
2. Flex to elbow to 90°
3. Whilst pressing on the radial head, supinate the forearm
4. A palpable click confirms reduction
5. In many cases the child will be using the arm within a few minutes
6. Child can be allowed home providing full supination pronation can be achieved
7. Advise parents to return in unlikely event that child is not using arm fully in 24 hours

8. Use of sling is discretionary – the child will use arm when ready
9. Ensure parents have supply of paracetamol at home
10. Advise about how caused and how to avoid in the future. All parents lift their children by the wrists, but tell them they must avoid for next few weeks and minimize until age of five years.

Scaphoid fracture

KEY POINTS

- At initial presentation, the diagnosis is clinical
- The radial nerve runs over the anatomical snuff box and is tender when compressed, therefore compare both sides. The diagnosis needs more than just ASB tenderness
- Clinical diagnosis warrants immobilization
- It is unusual in children.

ASSESSMENT

1. Usually results from a fall on the outstretched hand or other hyperextension injuries
2. Scaphoid fracture gives tenderness in anatomical snuff box, over scaphoid anteriorly and on axial compression of thumb towards radius
3. Pain on pincer grip of thumb against the index finger
4. Pain with ulnar deviation of the wrist
5. Request scaphoid views, not wrist.

MANAGEMENT

1. Fracture visible on X-ray
   - scaphoid POP cast
   - high arm sling
   - analgesia
2. Fracture not visible
   - Treatment is controversial. There is no evidence that delay in diagnosis changes prognosis
   - treat as for fracture
3. Established non-union
   - may present as new injury
   - discuss with orthopaedic surgeon – may wish to undertake fixation with grafting
4. Follow-up according to local policy.

Smoke inhalation

KEY POINTS

- A well patient can deteriorate very rapidly
- History is important in predicting those with an airway at risk
- Early intervention is required in high risk cases
- Think of other toxic agents which may have been inhaled
- Pulse oximetry may be misleading. The machine cannot differentiate oxyhaemoglobin from carboxyhaemoglobin.

ASSESSMENT

1. Detailed history of exposure – high risk includes confined space, trapped, prolonged exposure, toxic substances. Fire brigade may have important information
2. High risk symptoms – dyspnoea, wheeze, stridor, mucosal irritation, persistent cough, sooty sputum
3. High risk signs – hoarse voice, decreased conscious level, soot or burns in airway, burnt nostril hairs, peri-oral burns
4. High risk past medical history – COPD, asthma requiring regular treatment, other major respiratory disease
5. Send arterial blood gases, including carboxyhaemoglobin (metabolic acidosis – think of either missed hypovolaemia or cyanide inhalation)
6. Look for other injuries, e.g. due to blast, secondary missiles
7. Chest X-ray is rarely of use in initial assessment.

INDICATORS OF NEED FOR FURTHER INVESTIGATION/ASSESSMENT

1. Anyone with high risk features will need admission and observation
2. If any respiratory distress, stridor or hoarseness, summon

anaesthetist urgently or transfer immediately to suitable facility

3. Abnormal blood gases or carboxyhaemoglobin.

MANAGEMENT

1. Give 100% oxygen during assessment
2. Give nebulized salbutamol if bronchospasm.

If no high risk symptoms

1. Observe for one hour; if observations satisfactory and no new symptoms developed; can be supervised at home for next 24 hours
2. Return if develops new symptoms
3. Return as emergency if hoarse voice, short of breath, stridor develops
4. See GP if any persisting respiratory symptoms after 48 hours.

Sprained thumb

- Mechanism of injury varies and may help identify structure damaged
- Rupture of ulnar-collateral ligament of the metacarpophalangeal joint (MCPJ) of the thumb occurs in abduction injuries, e.g. dry slope skiing
- Swelling is often marked with soft tissue injuries and limits movement.

ASSESSMENT

1. Ask about mechanism of injury and area of maximum pain
2. Look for the distribution of any swelling, bruise, and restriction of movements
3. Palpate the thumb for tenderness paying particular attention to the collateral ligaments of the MCPJ
4. Check for laxity by comparing with the unaffected side.
5. Assess for bony tenderness especially in the anatomical snuffbox.

INDICATORS OF NEED FOR FURTHER INVESTIGATION/ASSESSMENT

Patients with rupture of the ulnar collateral ligament should be referred to orthopaedic surgeons for consideration of surgical repair.

MANAGEMENT

If X-rays normal and no laxity:
1. Advise simple analgesia, gentle exercise and elevation
2. Apply a high arm sling to reduce swelling
3. Support can be provided with an elastoplast or splint thumb spica for one week initially.

Subungual haematoma

- Crush injury
- Severe pain caused by pressure of blood trapped under nail.

ASSESSMENT

1. Examination – blood visible under the nail
2. X-ray – to exclude bony injury which will be technically compound if trephined.

TREATMENT

1. Trephining using heated needle or paper clip
2. Antibiotics if fracture present.

Support of injured limb

KEY POINTS

- Various methods of supporting injured limbs are available
- Advise patients to exercise those joints not immobilized
- Injury or immobilization of one part puts extra strain on other parts. Ensure that patients can manage daily tasks safely and are given advice on minimizing the effect on non-injured parts.

BROAD ARM SLING

1. Uses a triangular bandage to support the upper arm and elbow
2. The elbow should be flexed to slightly more than 90°, avoiding the hand becoming dependent and swollen
3. The sling takes the weight of the arm
4. Advise the patient to remove the sling to exercise uninjured parts regularly.

HIGH ARM SLING

1. Uses a triangular bandage to elevate the forearm, wrist and hand
2. The hand should be positioned with fingertips at the opposite shoulder
3. Patients find these slings difficult to reapply. The hand has a tendency to drop from under the sling causing pressure at the wrist. A modified broad arm sling is easier to reapply
4. Used mainly to reduce or prevent swelling of the wrist and hand. The sling should be worn when the patient is up and about, but in most cases can be removed and the arm elevated on cushions when resting.

COLLAR AND CUFF

1. Uses a foam covered strip secured around the neck and wrist to support the arm
2. The weight of the arm is not supported at the elbow, therefore useful for conditions where gravity helps to maintain fracture position and comfort
3. The elbow should be flexed slightly more than 90° to prevent the hand becoming dependent and swollen.

TUBIGRIP

1. A tubular elasticated bandage used to provide support and control swelling, although there is little evidence to support either role
2. Should extend towards the joints above and below the injured area, e.g. for knee, from mid thigh to above ankle
3. Beware constriction if the bandage rolls down (especially on the thigh)
4. Should be removed at night.

PLASTER OF PARIS BACKSLABS

1. Provide additional support and immobilization
2. Used for some soft tissue injuries as well as fractures
3. Apply tubular gauze next to the skin, followed by a layer of padding
4. POP slabs applied to 50–75% limb circumference and held in place with bandage
5. Not circumferential, therefore allow for swelling
6. Any period of immobilization is followed by some stiffness; this is worse the longer the period of immobilization
7. The weight of the cast can cause discomfort
8. Requires additional support for at least 48 hours, e.g. sling, crutches
9. Patients should be given plaster instructions (p. 81).

THUMB SPICA

1. Usually elastoplast; bandage slips and has little effect
2. Very itchy
3. Offers some support for sprained thumb
4. Commercial, removable splints are available and are more convenient but more expensive.

STRAPPING

1. Many techniques available to support or control ligament/tendon injuries
2. Specialist skill
3. Used mainly in sports injuries.

Temporomandibular joint dislocation

KEY POINTS

- May cause airway problem, especially if patient vomits, so ensure suction available
- Think of drug induced dystonia.

ASSESSMENT

1. Occurs following yawning, laughing, chewing hard
2. Characterized by sudden onset of severe pain, inability to close mouth and protrusion of the jaw
3. Usually bilateral. If unilateral, chin deviates away from dislocation.

INDICATORS OF NEED FOR FURTHER INVESTIGATION/ASSESSMENT

1. Suspicion of associated fracture (e.g. history of trauma)
2. Failure to reduce
3. Admit if consciousness level or gag reflex reduced, e.g. associated head injury, alcohol induced, following analgesia.

MANAGEMENT

1. X-ray before reduction if history of trauma
2. Always have suction available as patient may have difficulty expelling oral contents (e.g. after vomiting)
3. Do not undertake this technique in the drunk or unco-operative patient, who may be inclined to bite you
4. Give intramuscular or intravenous analgesia (recurrent dislocations may not require this)

5. Put on surgical gloves and wrap thumbs with gauze
6. Position yourself above the patient, e.g. patient sitting and you standing
7. Place thumbs onto lower molars, index fingers behind ramus and other fingers beneath jaw
8. Push downwards with gradually increasing force
9. The TMJ should be felt to relocate
10. Beware of patient yawning as sedation lightens
11. Arrange X-ray to confirm relocation
12. Refer to maxillofacial surgeon for follow-up
13. Soft diet until review
14. Oral analgesia.

ALTERNATIVE

1. Sedate as above
2. Touch back of throat with tongue depressor. Gagging may cause reduction of the dislocation.

Medical conditions that present at minor injuries units

Acute atraumatic back pain

KEY POINTS

- Check carefully for a history of trauma
- Most cases do not require X-ray
- Most are relieved by analgesia
- Early mobilization is recommended.

ASSESSMENT

1. Nature of pain; precipitating factors, relieving factors, diurnal variation
2. Neurological symptoms and signs – always ask about bladder and bowel dysfunction
3. Check for breast and prostatic malignancy
4. Assess swelling, tenderness, back movement
5. Gait
6. Straight leg raising and neurological assessment of lower limbs
7. Always do rectal examination to evaluate tone and assess perineal sensation.

UNFAVOURABLE FEATURES

Fever, weight loss, rest pain, lack of past problems in older person, not relieved with bed rest, motor or sensory symptoms, bladder or bowel dysfunction, bony tenderness.

INDICATORS OF NEED FOR X-RAY

1. Suspicion of malignancy
2. Suspicion of infection, including TB
3. Presence of unfavourable features
4. Failing to resolve despite adequate conservative treatment
5. Children and the elderly
6. Pain for more than six weeks despite treatment

MANAGEMENT OF SIMPLE MECHANICAL PAIN

1. Adequate analgesia – combine regular ibuprofen with an analgesic, e.g. Co-proxamol
2. Initial rest for 12–48 hours
3. Mobilize as early as possible
4. Physiotherapy or advice on exercise regime
5. Advise on posture and lifting
6. Occupational advice
7. Review by GP if not resolved in five days
8. If minor neurological signs, then treat as above and arrange review in 12–24 hours. Tell patient to contact GP if symptoms worsen, or any bowel or bladder symptoms.

If sinister features:
1. Treat as for simple mechanical pain
2. Arrange urgent outpatient appointment for further investigation
3. Admit if neurological symptoms/signs deteriorate, or if pain not resolving
4. Tell patient to contact urgently if pain worsens or bladder/bowel symptoms.

Admit if:
1. Cord compression
2. Severe pain
3. Unable to cope at home due to immobility etc.

ACUTE CORD COMPRESSION

Suggested by weakness, altered sensation, bladder or bowel dysfunction, altered tone and reflexes, lax sphincters, sensory level.

Action Needs emergency referral.

Acute gout

KEY POINTS

- Consider in all cases of hot, red, painful joint
- More frequent in middle-aged and elderly
- Classically affects the metatarsophalangeal joint of the big toe, but can affect any synovial joint.

ASSESSMENT

1. Ask about previous episodes, trauma, infection. Note drugs and other precipitating factors
2. The joint is warm, red, swollen and extremely tender with reduced movement
3. Inspect carefully for signs of soft tissue infection; blisters, breaks in the skin, ascending infection, increased temperature
4. Look at other joints for signs of inflammation, new or old.

INDICATORS OF NEED FOR FURTHER INVESTIGATION/ASSESSMENT

1. X-rays in the acute phase will show little change
2. Differential diagnosis with septic arthritis may be difficult. Septic joints tend to be immobile and the patient toxic. If in doubt arrange further investigation
3. Blood can be taken for urate levels, although the best diagnostic test is examination of joint fluid which should be aspirated under aseptic technique.

MANAGEMENT

1. Advise rest and elevation until the acute inflammation has settled
2. Indomethacin or other nonsteroidal is best anti-inflamma-

tory. If contraindicated, try paracetamol or codeine/paracetamol mix for pain relief
3. Advise patient to reattend/seek help if there is failure to resolve, worsening pain or stiffness, fever or malaise.

Acute paronychia

- A soft tissue infection adjacent to the nail, commonly caused by *Staphylococcus aureus*
- Early stages may present as only erythema and pain, that precede abscess formation
- Can be presentation or complication of diabetes mellitus.

ASSESSMENT

1. Check for local spread to pulp and bone (indicated by swelling of pulp as well as dorsal aspect)
2. Check for spreading infection (lymphangitis, lymphadenopathy, temperature)
3. Capillary blood sugar measurement.

INDICATORS OF NEED FOR FURTHER INVESTIGATION/ASSESSMENT

1. X-ray if:
   - evidence of bony involvement, to exclude osteomyelitis
   - possibility of foreign body
   - failing to resolve despite adequate antibiotics
2. Elevated capillary blood sugar needs further investigation.

MANAGEMENT

1. Erythema only
   - give flucloxacillin (or erythromycin if allergic to penicillin)
   - analgesia
   - advise elevation
   - return if worsens or not improved in 48 hours

2. Abscess present
   - incise under local anaesthetic ring block
   - antibiotics are not routinely required
3. If cellulitis spreading proximal to distal interphalangeal joint, incise and give antibiotics.

ALTERNATIVES

Another acceptable form of management is to gently insert a blunt probe under the cuticular fold into the abscess cavity. With a significant sized abscess this can be achieved without local anaesthetic.

Analgesia

KEY POINTS

- Pain is the commonest reason for emergency presentation
- Early relief of pain is not only humanitarian, it speeds recovery
- Never forget the importance of reassurance
- Physical support of an injury or reduction of a dislocation are important means of relieving pain.

PRINCIPLES

1. Acute severe pain needs intravenous analgesia
2. Intravenous analgesia should be given as a large diluted volume (10–20 ml) titrated against effect
3. Analgesics do not mask hard clinical signs, e.g. peritonism, and invariably make examination easier.

THE SPECTRUM OF ANALGESIA

Aspirin, paracetamol
Co-proxamol, Co-dydramol
codeine, dihydrocodeine
opioid analgesics

Increasing pain

NONSTEROIDAL ANALGESICS

These provide useful pain relief for musculoskeletal pain, although they are inappropriate for major fractures. Their use is limited by side effects, in particular gastrointestinal bleeding and exacerbation of asthma. In the elderly they may cause fluid retention.

They are most frequently used as oral preparations. Topical gel form is widely marketed but its value is disputed.

103

Intramuscular nonsteroidals are now widely used and are useful for the treatment of renal colic and avoid the use of opiates. They have the same diagnostic indications as oral NSAIDs, they are not a replacement for intramuscular opiates and should not be used in chest and abdominal pain. Suppositories are also available and are as effective as intramuscular analgesia.

GASEOUS ANALGESIA

Nitrous oxide mixed with oxygen (50:50) is a good fast short-acting analgesic. It is contraindicated in chest injury, head injury, decompression sickness and early after abdominal surgery.

LOCAL ANAESTHESIA (q.v.)

This provides excellent pain relief and is most widely used in limb injuries. Either local infiltration or regional techniques can be used. Remember to record the sensation in the area before administering local anaesthetic.

ICE, ELEVATION AND GENTLE EXERCISE

This regime is excellent for the relief of pain from soft tissue swelling and can be combined with other forms of analgesia.

Ice can be applied in two ways:
1. An ice cube can be moved over the affected area with a continuous movement to stop local ice burns. Oil can be put on the skin before the ice to help this
2. Ice or a bag of frozen peas can be wrapped in a moist cotton towel and held on the area for 5–10 minutes.

Following the ice application, undertake gentle exercises.

IMMOBILIZATION

The pain of musculoskeletal injuries is reduced by immobilization. However, prolonged immobilization can lead to stiffness and muscle wasting.

Antitetanus prophylaxis*

KEY POINTS

- All wounds or breaks in the skin are sources of entry for tetanus
- This includes burns.

Immunization status	Type of wound	Type of wound
	Clean	Tetanus prone
Last of three dose course, or reinforcing dose within last 10 years	Nil	Nil (a dose of human tetanus immuno-globulin may be given if risk of infection is considered especially high, e.g. contamination with stable manure)
Last of three dose course or reinforcing dose more than 10 years previously	A reinforcing dose of adsorbed vaccine	A reinforcing dose of adsorbed vaccine plus a dose of human tetanus immunoglobulin
Not immunized or immunization status not known with certainty	A full three dose course of adsorbed vaccine	A full three dose course of vaccine, plus a dose of tetanus immunoglobulin in a different site

1. The prophylaxis dose of human tetanus immunoglobulin is 250 i.u. by intramuscular injection. It should be given at a different site to the absorbed vaccine
2. A full course of absorbed vaccine consists of three doses at intervals of one month
3. Corneal abrasions require tetanus prophylaxis as for any other wound

4. For immunized adults, who have received five doses, either in childhood or as an adult, booster doses are not recommended *except* in tetanus prone wounds.

The following are considered tetanus prone wounds:
1. Any wound or burn over six hours old before treatment
2. Wounds or burns of any age if:
   - significant degree of devitalized tissue
   - puncture type wounds
   - contact with soil or manure
   - clinical evidence of infection.

NB Thorough cleansing of wound is essential regardless of tetanus immunization status.

CONTRAINDICATIONS TO TETANUS VACCINE

1. Acute febrile illness
2. History of anaphylaxis to previous dose.

REFERENCE

Immunisation Against Infectious Disease, HMSO 1996.

* Adapted from *Immunisation Against Infectious Disease*, HMSO, 1996. © Crown copyright. Reproduced with the permission of the Controller of Her Majesty's Stationery Office.

Arc eye

KEY POINTS

- Presents several hours after exposure to ultraviolet radiation, e.g. welding or using a sun bed without adequate eye protection
- Watering, pain and redness affects both eyes
- Pain and blephorospasm are prominent features.

ASSESSMENT

Local anaesthetic eye drops provide immediate relief of symptoms and allow full examination of the eye. As they inhibit corneal reflexes they should only be used to allow examination, not for treatment.

INDICATORS OF NEED FOR FURTHER INVESTIGATION/ASSESSMENT

Persistence of symptoms for more than 24 hours.

MANAGEMENT

1. Provide oral analgesia
2. Topical antibiotics help to prevent infection of the damaged corneal epithelium
3. A firm eye pad may give symptomatic relief but should not be applied to both eyes, rendering the patient blind.

ALTERNATIVES

Other acceptable forms of management include:

In addition to treatment above, mydriatic eye drops (e.g. cyclopentalate 1%) will dilate the pupil and relieve pain. Patients must be advised not to drive for one to two hours.

Asthma inhaler requests

KEY POINTS

- Out of hours or A&E requests for inhaler replacement are usually due to worsening symptoms which have led to increased inhaler use and therefore unexpected 'running out'
- These are not quick cases but require full assessment, as for any asthmatic patient.

ASSESSMENT

1. All patients should be assessed and treated according to British Thoracic Society asthma care guidelines
2. Take a full history. Examine the patient recording pulse, blood pressure, respiratory rate and peak expiratory flow rate. Look for signs of severe or life-threatening asthma.

INDICATORS OF NEED FOR FURTHER INVESTIGATION/ASSESSMENT

PEFR <75% or deterioration during management requires more aggressive therapy, initially with nebulized bronchodilator.

MANAGEMENT

1. If PEFR >75% predicted or best, give inhaled bronchodilator
2. Observe for 60 minutes, if the patient is stable and PEFR is >75% the patient may be discharged with a replacement inhaler
3. Check inhaler technique and advise early review with their GP
4. Advise the patient to return/seek help if symptoms worsen.

Bell's facial palsy

KEY POINTS

- Other causes of facial palsy must be excluded
- Early high dose prednisolone is of value.

DIFFERENTIAL DIAGNOSIS

1. Intracranial
   - acoustic neuroma
   - brain stem tumour
   - meningitis
   - multiple sclerosis
   - polio
   - stroke
2. Intra temporal
   - cholesteatoma
   - otitis media
   - Ramsay Hunt syndrome
3. Infra temporal
   - parotid tumour
   - trauma
4. Others
   - diabetes
   - Guillain-Barré syndrome
   - Lyme disease
   - sarcoid.

ASSESSMENT

1. Sudden onset of facial weakness and asymmetry
2. May have associated pain, in particular in the post auricular region
3. Bell's palsy is a lower motor neurone palsy, i.e. unilateral weakness including forehead

4. Sagging mouth, drooling, taste impairment
5. Inability to close eye, watering of eye or dry eye
6. Exclude other cranial nerve signs and signs of raised intracranial pressure
7. Examine ears and parotid.

INDICATORS OF NEED FOR FURTHER INVESTIGATION/ASSESSMENT

1. Upper motor neurone facial palsy
2. History of trauma
3. Evidence of infection, including herpes zoster
4. Any symptoms or signs beyond the facial nerve.

MANAGEMENT

1. If within four days of onset give 40–80 mg prednisolone daily for one week
2. Hypromellose eye drops four hourly and eye protection if cornea remains exposed on closing eyelids. Consider eye pad for few days
3. Review in four to five days.

AFTERCARE

1. Advise on reversible nature
2. Reassure this is not a stroke
3. Return if new signs or symptoms develop
4. Variable time course from days to months
5. Consider ENT referral if not settling rapidly, to exclude other causes.

Bites

Animal bites

- Wound infection is the most significant complication
- Rabies is not endemic in UK, but patients may present following bites abroad.

ASSESSMENT

1. History of the event including animal, time elapsed etc.
2. Examination as for any wound.

MANAGEMENT

1. Ensure adequate anaesthesia
2. Thorough cleaning and irrigation of wound
3. Tetanus immunization as appropriate
4. Dressing
5. Antibiotic – amoxycillin
6. Review in two to three days and consider delayed primary closure
7. Rabies immunization if required (can be given up to a few weeks after patient exposure).

ALTERNATIVES

1. For cosmetic reasons facial wounds may be sutured but only after thorough cleaning
2. Consider plastic surgery referral
3. Puncture wounds should never be closed.

Human bites

- High incidence of infection
- Hepatitis B may be transmitted
- HIV has been isolated in saliva, but there is no documentation of transmission through bites
- Injuries sustained to hand by punching someone on the teeth should be treated as bites
- Remember that most tongue cuts are self-inflicted bites.

ASSESSMENT

1. As for other bites
2. Look for teeth in wound, especially hand wounds.

MANAGEMENT

1. Thorough cleaning
2. Tetanus immunization as appropriate
3. Leave wounds open unless cosmetically unacceptable
4. Co-amoxiclav is the antibiotic of choice (to cover against anaerobes)
5. Elevate as necessary
6. Advise on exercises.

Insect bites

KEY POINTS

- Often difficult to differentiate between local allergic reaction and infection
- Beware risk of anaphylaxis.

ASSESSMENT

1. Nature of wound
2. Look for evidence of infection.

MANAGEMENT

1. Tetanus immunization as appropriate
2. Antihistamine for allergic component (topical is often sufficient)
3. Cold compress provides symptomatic relief
4. Antibiotics if evidence of cellulitis
5. Elevate injured part if possible.

Bleeding tooth socket

Presents as a complication after tooth extraction. The bleeding is from the alveolar mucosa, which may be torn, rather than from the socket itself.

KEY POINTS

- Dentists should provide 24 hour cover for their patients, and patients should be advised that this is their first port of call
- Significant blood loss may occur if bleeding is allowed to continue, therefore careful assessment of the control of bleeding should be made and further referral may be required.

ASSESSMENT

Check for risk factors which may complicate management, such as anticoagulant therapy.

INDICATORS OF NEED FOR FURTHER INVESTIGATION/ASSESSMENT

If the measures below fail to control the bleeding, referral to a dental surgeon should be arranged.

MANAGEMENT

1. Remove loose blood clot
2. Roll a piece of gauze and place it over the socket; instruct the patient to bite onto this for 10 minutes
3. If this does not control bleeding, pack the socket with an alginate dressing, top with rolled gauze and bite again for 10 minutes.

ALTERNATIVES

Other acceptable forms of management include inserting a horizontal mattress suture across the socket under local anaesthetic, top with a gauze roll and bite for 10 minutes.

Bleeding varicose veins

KEY POINTS

- Often profuse bleeding from a comparatively trivial injury
- May occur spontaneously.

ASSESSMENT

1. Check pulse and blood pressure
2. Examine wound and confirm underlying varicose veins.

MANAGEMENT

1. Elevate limb
2. Apply pressure for at least five minutes
3. IV fluids as required, depending on clinical situation
4. Once bleeding is under control, treat the wound as appropriate
5. Most occur in the pretibial area in elderly patients and should not be sutured.

ADVICE TO PATIENTS

1. Instruct on first aid measures in case it occurs again
2. If required – elective surgical referral for definitive management.

INDICATIONS FOR REFERRAL

1. Failure to control bleeding
2. Shock
3. Recurrent episodes
4. Patient lives alone.

Button cell battery ingestion

KEY POINTS

- Some batteries have toxic doses of mercury
- Batteries are corroded by stomach acid
- Batteries can corrode mucosa because of electric current produced.

ASSESSMENT

1. Determine type of battery – contact National Poisons Information Service (p. 143)
2. Examine oropharynx
3. Check for signs of oesophageal perforation, e.g. surgical emphysema
4. Check for abdominal signs
5. Ensure no evidence of mercury poisoning – excessive salivation, nausea, vomiting, tremor, abnormal behaviour.

All cases need X-ray to determine the location of the battery – undertake plain chest and abdomen X-rays with shielding of gonads.

MANAGEMENT

Needs surgical intervention if signs of perforation.

1. Battery in pharynx/oesophagus:
   - A drink may move battery into the stomach. Give one drink and then re-X-ray. Do not give large drink as may need anaesthetic later
   - Endoscopic removal
2. Battery in stomach:
   - Re-X-ray in 24 hours if battery intact

- If still in stomach after 24 hours then remove endoscopically.
- Some advise giving cisapride to help gastric emptying
- Some advise giving antacids or anti-acid drugs to decrease corrosion of battery

3. Battery beyond stomach:
   - Reassure if intact. Return if symptomatic
   - Re-X-ray in two to three days. If no signs of progress, refer for removal

4. Battery not intact:
   - If seen as fragmented on X-ray, blurred edges on X-ray or broken on removal, check blood mercury levels and seek advise of NPIS.

AFTERCARE

Give advice on storage of batteries and other ingestable products, e.g. medicines.

Cold sores

KEY POINTS

- Herpes simplex infection
- Immunosuppressed patients can have widespread ulcers and difficulty drinking
- Tingling sensation precedes blisters.

ASSESSMENT

1. Check lesion is well localized
2. Check for evidence of immunosuppression
3. Check for triggers, e.g. stress, intercurrent illness
4. Presents as tingling, blistering lesion on lip or inside mouth.

INDICATORS OF NEED FOR FURTHER INVESTIGATION/ASSESSMENT

1. Pronounced fever
2. Extensive oral vesicles
3. Difficulty swallowing.

MANAGEMENT

1. Best treated when tingling present, before rash appears
2. Topical acyclovir if within 48 hours of rash appearance (contraindicated in pregnancy)
3. Avoid contact with young babies and immunosuppressed patients until lesion dry.

Conjunctivitis

KEY POINTS

- Itchy, gritty, watering or sticky red eye
- Uncomfortable rather than painful – pain as the predominant symptom suggests other diagnoses.

ASSESSMENT

1. Ask about duration and type of symptoms, any treatment already used, exposure to chemicals or light (see arc eye, p. 108) previous episodes and other medical conditions
2. A complete examination of the eye including visual acuity, lid eversion and fluorescein staining should be carried out
3. The conjunctiva appears red and inflamed
4. Mucopurulent discharge may be present.

INDICATORS OF NEED FOR FURTHER INVESTIGATION/ASSESSMENT

1. Failure to respond to topical treatment
2. Reduced visual acuity
3. Corneal ulceration or fluorescein staining
4. Subconjunctival haemorrhage (haemorrhagic conjunctivitis caused by enterovirus)
5. Pain as main symptom.

MANAGEMENT

1. Advise careful hygiene; conjunctivitis is contagious
2. Prescribe topical chloramphenicol or fucidic acid
3. Bathe the eye with water to remove discharge
4. Advise patient to return/seek help if symptoms not improved in 24–48 hours.

Continued epistaxis

KEY POINTS

- Often due to inadequate pressure technique
- Always check blood pressure
- Think of clotting disorders and poor anticoagulant control
- In the elderly rapidly leads to hypovolaemic shock
- Wear eye and face protection when examining and treating.

ASSESSMENT

1. Check pulse, capillary refill and blood pressure
2. History or signs of bleeding problems
3. Drug history, e.g. warfarin, aspirin
4. Check clotting if history suggests potential problem or if bleeding does not stop with simple measures
5. With suction available: using nasal speculae inspect nostrils for source of bleeding
6. Cotton wool bud soaked with 1 in 1000 adrenaline may aid this.

MANAGEMENT

If clinically shocked or major blood loss seen (>500 ml)
1. Lie person on side
2. Get patient to squeeze firmly over the cartilaginous portion of the nose and breathe through mouth
3. Tell them to spit any blood from mouth into a bowl, not to swallow it
4. Establish venous access and take blood for FBC, grouping, clotting studies
5. Commence volume replacement
6. Proceed with techniques below to stop bleeding

7. Speak to ENT surgeon whilst preparing to undertake this.

If not clinically shocked – anterior bleeding
1. Sit person leaning forwards
2. Get patient to squeeze firmly over the cartilaginous portion of the nose and breathe through mouth
3. Tell them to spit any blood from mouth into a bowl, not to swallow it
4. Apply ice pack to bridge of nose/glabellar region
5. Continue applying pressure for 10 minutes as timed on a clock
   • if stopped, observe for 20 minutes before allowing home
   • if continuing loss, cauterize well-localized bleeding point with silver nitrate stick. Wet the stick before use then roll over the area for about 10 seconds. Only ever cauterize one side of septum, and only a small area. Or use anterior nasal pack/nasal tampon, and arrange ENT appointment
6. Refer to ENT specialist if these are not successful.

If not clinically shocked – posterior bleeding
1. Position patient as suggested above
2. Insert a well lubricated 12 Foley catheter through the nostril
3. Pass until seen in throat or gagging is induced
4. Inflate balloon
5. Pull back until balloon impacts in posterior nasal space
6. Secure to cheek with tape under slight tension
7. Insert an anterior nasal pack/tampon
8. Both sides may need occluding
9. Refer to ENT surgeon.

INDICATORS OF NEED FOR FURTHER INVESTIGATION/ASSESSMENT
1. Posterior nasal bleeding

2. Failure to control bleeding
3. Abnormal clotting
4. Uncontrolled hypertension
5. Pack *in situ*.

AFTERCARE

If bleeding stopped and allowed home:
1. Do not blow nose for 48 hours, dab it with soft handkerchief
2. Do not pick nose or try to clean with cotton wool
3. Do not sniff hard
4. Return if bleeding restarts and does not stop with 10 minutes of pressure.
5. Re-instruct on technique of pinching cartilaginous portion of nose.

Earache (non-traumatic)

KEY POINTS

- Think of local causes and referred pain
- Local causes include barotrauma, bullous myringitis, mastoiditis, otitis externa (p. 144), otitis media
- Referred pain may be from teeth, cervical nodes, cervical spine, facial nerve or throat.

ASSESSMENT

1. Barotrauma will occur after flying or diving – conductive deafness with middle ear effusion
2. Blisters on drum or in canal in bullous myringitis
3. Evidence of mastoiditis – fever, hearing loss, foul discharge, pain behind ear, swelling behind ear and pain on movement of ear
4. Inflamed ear drum with fever suggests otitis media.

INDICATORS OF NEED FOR FURTHER INVESTIGATION/ASSESSMENT

1. Acute mastoiditis
2. Cholesteatoma
3. Associated facial palsy.

MANAGEMENT

1. Otitis media – amoxycillin, decongestants, analgesia, aural toilet if required
2. Otitis externa – see p. 144
3. Barotrauma – analgesia, decongestants, advise on avoidance in future
4. Bullous myringitis often requires no treatment, but acyclovir if herpetic infection.

Emergency contraception

- Hormonal emergency contraception must be started within 72 hours of intercourse
- An intrauterine device can be used to provide postcoital contraception up to five days after calculated earliest day of ovulation.

ASSESSMENT

1. Exclude pregnancy
2. Check blood pressure
3. Hormonal emergency contraception is indicated within 72 hours of unprotected intercourse, accidents with barrier contraception or if one or more oral contraceptive pill has been missed at the start or end or the pill-free interval, making it longer than seven days
4. It is contraindicated in pregnancy, after recent thromboembolic event, or when migraine with neurological disturbance is present at the time of request. Previous ectopic pregnancy is a relative contraindication

INDICATORS OF NEED FOR FURTHER INVESTIGATION/ASSESSMENT

If a normal period does not follow or is lighter or shorter than usual, emergency contraception may not have been effective and pregnancy must be excluded.

MANAGEMENT

1. Prescribe PC4 as per *BNF*, in two doses 12 hours apart.
2. Advise follow-up to discuss future contraception.

Fish bone in throat

KEY POINTS

- Bones may cause a mucosal tear which gives sensation of a persistent foreign body
- Any bone in respiratory tract or oesophagus needs removal.

ASSESSMENT

1. Ask about type of fish – e.g. cod have larger bones, red mullet bones are relatively radiolucent
2. What has patient drunk or eaten since pain started?
3. Dysphagia, salivation, constant pain suggest impaction. This is supported by inability to swallow a test drink
4. Any coughing or respiratory distress suggests inhalation.

INDICATORS OF NEED FOR FURTHER INVESTIGATION/ASSESSMENT

1. Inability to remove fish bone
2. Dysphagia, drooling, significant symptoms.

MANAGEMENT

1. If visible in pharynx, especially tonsils, then remove under direct vision
2. If not distressed and able to swallow fluids and solids with normal examination, then can be discharged with advice to return if symptoms worsen or fail to resolve in 24 hours.

Fits in known epileptics

KEY POINTS

- Epileptics will occasionally have fits
- Major fits are often associated with subtherapeutic drug levels
- Most epileptics who have fits do not require admission.

ASSESSMENT AFTER FIT COMPLETE

1. Check for persisting neurological signs
2. Ensure fully alert and orientated
3. Check for injuries, especially to head
4. Verify medication and whether any recent change or omissions or reason for poor absorption
5. Check for precipitating factors, including alcohol, hypoglycaemia, strobe lights.

MANAGEMENT

Immediate management
1. Protect patient from injury, e.g. protect head, remove or pad sharp objects
2. Put person in recovery position if possible
3. Clear airway
4. Do not restrain
5. Confirm they are known to be epileptic
6. Reassure bystanders, stop others from rushing in to help.

Continued fitting
1. Consider other diagnoses, e.g. hypoglycaemia, head injury, eclampsia
2. Give oxygen if possible
3. Administer diazepam intravenously or per rectum

Prolonged fitting
1. Give oxygen
2. Further intravenous diazepam emulsion
3. Second line anti-epileptic agent, e.g. phenytoin, chlormethiazole.

All cases
1. Check serum anti-convulsant levels unless single short-lived fit
2. Search for cause of fit, e.g. drug compliance, alcohol ingestion, drug interaction.

INDICATIONS FOR ADMISSION

1. Incomplete recovery
2. Prolonged fitting
3. Atypical fit
4. Increased number of fits.

CRITERIA FOR DISCHARGE HOME

Must satisfy the following criteria:
1. Full recovery from fit
2. Supervision for next 24 hours
3. Absence of head injury.

AFTERCARE

Before discharge home:
1. Check for precipitating factors and give appropriate advice
2. Advise to see GP for blood results
3. Check on occupation and driving status, especially if first daytime fit.

Foreign bodies in nose and ear

Usually small objects in small children!

KEY POINTS

- Attempts at removal should only be made if the object and surrounding structures can be clearly seen, in order to prevent further injury
- Avoid multiple attempts with inadequate equipment. Most foreign bodies in the nose and ear can be left *in situ* until the patient can be seen by an ENT surgeon
- Button batteries can leak and cause tissue necrosis; they should be removed as soon as possible.

ASSESSMENT

1. Assess for airway compromise with a foreign body in the nose (very rare)
2. Attempt to visualize the object and make an assessment of the likely cooperation of the patient.

INDICATORS OF NEED FOR FURTHER INVESTIGATION/ASSESSMENT

1. Airway compromise
2. Dysphagia or drooling
3. Refer to ENT those patients in whom you cannot remove the object.

MANAGEMENT

1. Live insects in the ear can be killed and floated out by filling the external auditory meatus with olive oil
2. Objects in the nose may be shifted by occluding the opposite nostril and asking the patient to blow sharply through their nose

3. Objects which can be visualized well and are within reach may be lifted out with fine forceps
4. Smooth surfaced objects should be pushed out by using a hook from behind, to avoid impacting the object.

Foreign body in the eye

These may be tiny dust particles or larger metal fragments. Patients may be unaware that a foreign body has entered the eye and is the cause of symptoms. Patients usually present with a sore, irritating red eye.

KEY POINTS

- Make a careful search for foreign bodies in any patient complaining of a sore or irritating eye
- Beware of penetrating foreign bodies more likely to occur during activities such as chiselling.

ASSESSMENT

1. Carry out a full examination of the eye, remembering to record visual acuity and to evert the eyelid in search of a subtarsal foreign body
2. Fluorescein eye drops will show up corneal abrasions. Multiple linear abrasions suggest a subtarsal foreign body.

INDICATORS OF NEED FOR FURTHER INVESTIGATION/ASSESSMENT

1. Reduced visual acuity
2. Corneal ulcer or large abrasion
3. Inability to remove the foreign body
4. Evidence of penetrating injury.

MANAGEMENT

1. If a slit lamp is not available, lie the patient flat with a good light source overhead
2. Instil short-acting local anaesthetic eye drops into the affected eye

3. If the foreign body is loose, remove it with irrigation or a cotton bud
4. If the foreign body is embedded or cannot be removed with the cotton bud, a needle may be used to lift it gently from the cornea
5. Treat any remaining defect in the cornea as an abrasion
6. If rust ring present, refer to ophthalmology clinic.

Gum infection

Dentists provide 24 hour cover.

ASSESSMENT

1. Abscess: severe toothache, pain on tapping tooth, local swelling of jaw area, high temperature
2. Gingivitis (gum infection): pain at base of tooth, bleeding from gums (especially after eating or brushing), foetor oris
3. Pericoronitis (infection around erupting or impacted tooth): pain may refer to ear, trismus, tender over gum
4. Assess for systemic illness
5. Assess for bleeding disorders as alternative cause.

INDICATORS OF NEED FOR FURTHER INVESTIGATION/ASSESSMENT

1. Evidence of apical or peri-apical abscess, refer to dentist/ dental unit at hospital
2. Systemically unwell.

MANAGEMENT

1. Amoxycillin for five days.
2. Metronidazole for five days
3. Analgesic
4. Antiseptic mouthwash after each meal
5. Return/attend dentist if worsening symptoms or not resolved when antibiotics complete
6. If fails to resolve, consider other causes or presence of abscess
7. Use as opportunity for dental care education and advise regular dental examination.

Headache

KEY POINT

There are many causes, but the majority are not significant.

ASSESSMENT

1. History
   - site
   - duration
   - frequency
   - nature
2. Associated features
   - visual disturbance
   - nausea/vomiting
   - neck pain
   - weakness
   - involuntary movements
3. Past history
   - trauma
   - drugs/alcohol
   - previous episodes
   - stress
4. Examination
   - check pulse/blood pressure
   - pupillary reaction
   - fundi
   - neurological
   - external examination of scalp
   - neck
   - sinuses.

MANAGEMENT

1. Patients with abnormal neurological signs will require urgent referral for investigation and management
2. Specific conditions will require specific management, e.g. sinusitis
3. The majority of patients will have no structural cause and require symptomatic analgesia and reassurance
4. Advise to return if worsens or develops new symptoms or signs.

Hypoglycaemia

KEY POINTS

- Any insulin-dependent diabetic who is confused, aggressive, drowsy or unconscious should be presumed to be hypoglycaemic
- Start treatment whilst checking capillary blood sugar
- Consider this in any patient with altered consciousness level
- May present as an acute neurological deficit.

ASSESSMENT

1. Clear airway and check gag reflex
2. Treat first
3. Look for injuries and causative factors.

CAUSES OF HYPOGLYCAEMIA IN NON-DIABETICS

1. Excessive alcohol
2. Insulinoma
3. Liver disease
4. Poisoning
5. Starvation/exhaustion.

INDICATORS OF NEED FOR FURTHER INVESTIGATION/ASSESSMENT

1. Failure to recover fully after treatment below
2. Non-diabetic patient
3. Does not satisfy criteria below in aftercare section
4. Hypoglycaemia due to sulphonylurea ingestion.

MANAGEMENT

Unconscious

Three treatments are available:
1. 1 mg glucagon either intramuscularly or subcutaneously. This may take up to 10 minutes to have full effect
2. Dextrose gel instilled in buccal sulcus with patient lying in recovery position
3. Dextrose intravenously. Flush with saline to reduce risk of thrombophlebitis.

NB Glucagon may be ineffective after prolonged hypoglycaemia and in non-diabetic hypoglycaemia.

Conscious
1. Ensure normal gag reflex is present
2. Give an oral source of glucose
   - sugary drink
   - dextrose tablets
   - dextrose gel
3. Improvement should occur within a few minutes. If it does not, reconsider diagnosis
4. Give source of starch, e.g. a sandwich
5. Find reason for hypoglycaemic attack and give appropriate advice to prevent further reccurence. Usual causes are unusual exercise, late or missed meal, change of insulin type or dose.

AFTERCARE

1. Can go home if
   - supervised for next 12 hours
   - full recovery
   - attack was not serious or unexplained
   - can manage to eat adequately (e.g. not due to vomiting)
2. Give appropriate advice and education.

Ingested/inhaled foreign body

KEY POINTS

- Any object in respiratory tract or oesophagus needs removal
- Once in stomach, most items pass harmlessly
- Button cell batteries need a different approach (p. 118).

ASSESSMENT

1. Dysphagia, salivation, retrosternal pain suggest oesophageal impaction. This is supported by inability to swallow a test drink
2. Any coughing, respiratory distress suggest inhalation
3. Look for signs of peritonitis
4. Most cases will need X-ray of chest
5. X-ray should include upper abdomen so that whole of oesophagus is included
6. Abdomen X-ray is not required
7. Only those with definite history of swallowing blunt object without coughing, respiratory problems, dysphagia or retrosternal pain can be safely reassured without X-ray.

MANAGEMENT

1. In pharynx or respiratory tract
   - if visible in pharynx, then remove under direct vision
   - refer for endoscopic removal
2. In oesophagus
   - discuss with surgeon before undertaking nonoperative treatment
   - simple drink may dislodge object
   - effervescent drink may be more successful but distends stomach (risk if anaesthesia required later)

- intravenous glucagon to augment oesophageal peristalsis (do not use for sharp objects)
- endoscopic removal

3. In stomach
   - reassure that object will pass if it is smooth-edged
   - no need to search stools for object (unless valuable)
   - if sharp-edged, referral for endoscopy
4. Beyond stomach
   - if smooth-edged, no treatment required
   - if sharp, consider admission and observation for evidence of perforation or surgical removal, depending on perceived risk
5. Normal diet
6. Return if develops any abdominal symptoms
7. May develop anal fissure when object passes.

National Poisons Information Services

TELEPHONE NUMBERS

Belfast	01232 240503
Birmingham	0121 507 5588
Cardiff	01222 709901
Dublin	+00353 (0)1 8379966
Edinburgh	0131 536 2300
Leeds	01132 430715
London	0171 635 9191
Newcastle	0191 232 5131

INFORMATION THEY WILL REQUIRE

1. Your name and telephone number
2. Patient's name and age
3. Substance ingested
   - trade name
   - generic/chemical name
   - manufacturer
4. Amount ingested; if uncertain, what is maximum possible
5. Medical and drug history of patient
6. Symptoms patient has experienced since ingestion
7. Clinical signs
8. Any treatment already given.

If tablet unidentifiable, then know:
1. Tablet or capsule
2. Colour of tablet
3. Shape
4. Scoring
4. Markings
6. Other identifiable features.

Otitis externa

KEY POINTS

- Often follows minor trauma from foreign objects in the ear
- Mixed bacterial growth.

ASSESSMENT

1. Pain worse with movement of pinna, chewing and yawning
2. May produce cellulitis anterior to the ear
3. Differentiate from well-localized feruncle in ear
4. Check for systemic symptoms and pyrexia
5. Discharge from ear often thick
6. Differential diagnoses of impetigo (when tends to spread over the ear) and herpetic infection (giving pain first and vesicle formation)
7. Check capillary blood sugar.

INDICATORS OF NEED FOR FURTHER INVESTIGATION/ASSESSMENT

1. Foreign body in ear
2. Large amount of discharge in external auditory canal, for suctioning.

MANAGEMENT

1. Clean ear canal by gentle syringing or cotton wool pledgets
2. Antibiotic ear drops every four hours
3. Oral flucloxacillin if spreading cellulitis, lymphadenopathy or pyrexia
4. Advice on prevention of further trauma to ear canal.

Panic attacks

KEY POINTS

- Acute onset of anxiety resulting in somatic symptoms and signs
- Always exclude other causes of high respiratory rate and tachycardia
- Explanation and reassurance are the most important part of treatment.

ASSESSMENT

1. Look for evidence of respiratory distress and signs of asthma
2. Check for dysrhythmias
3. Ensure no evidence of anaphylaxis, e.g. periorbital oedema, urticaria
4. Look for evidence of thyrotoxicosis
5. If in doubt, check arterial blood gases which will show a respiratory alkalosis in panic attack.

INDICATORS OF NEED FOR FURTHER INVESTIGATION/ASSESSMENT

Doubt regarding the diagnosis.

MANAGEMENT

1. Reassure the patient
2. Try to discover precipitating factor and remove it
3. Encourage rebreathing with a paper bag
4. If above fails and diagnosis is certain, then sedation may be required with an oral benzodiazepine
5. Educate about cause of the somatic symptoms

6. Explain about avoiding precipitating factors and relaxation techniques
7. Refer back to GP for long-term care, e.g. need for behavioural therapy, medication
8. Ensure not returning to source of stimulus.

Perforated ear drum

KEY POINTS

- Most heal spontaneously if infection is prevented
- If associated with head injury, needs admission.

ASSESSMENT

1. Assess pain from ear
2. Ensure that deafness is conductive
3. Carefully inspect external auditory meatus
4. Look for signs of fractured base of skull, e.g. battle sign, periorbital haematoma, epistaxis, rhinorrhoea, otorrhoea
5. If secondary to blast, check for other injuries including lung injury.

INDICATORS OF NEED FOR FURTHER INVESTIGATION/ASSESSMENT

1. If damage to inner ear is suspected
2. Associated with fractured base of skull.

MANAGEMENT

1. Amoxycillin 250 mg orally three times daily
2. Advise not to put anything in ear
3. Keep water out of ear, including no swimming
4. When showering put plug of cotton wool in outer ear – do not attempt to push down ear canal
5. Wipe away any external discharge but do not attempt to clean in ear canal
6. Seek medical help if pain worsens
7. Arrange ENT appointment by discussing with surgeon.

Phimosis and paraphimosis

KEY POINTS

- Phimosis occurs when the tight foreskin cannot be retracted over the glans. It may occur in association with balanitis. Rarely it can become so tight as to restrict urine flow, when circumcision may be required
- Paraphimosis occurs mainly in children or elderly men. The foreskin is retracted and forms a constricting ring leading to oedema, venous engorgement and ultimately gangrene of the glans
- Paraphimosis requires immediate reduction
- Analgesia or anaesthesia may be required. The procedures can be particularly distressing for a child, where recourse to general anaesthetic may be needed.

ASSESSMENT

1. Ask about onset, duration and previous episodes
2. Check urine flow
3. Check for signs of arterial compromise.

INDICATORS OF NEED FOR FURTHER INVESTIGATION/ASSESSMENT

1. Phimosis causing urinary retention should be referred to a urologist
2. Refer to urologist urgently if unable to reduce paraphimosis, or evidence of arterial compromise. Hyaluronidase injection or dorsal slit may be required to reduce the paraphimosis
3. All patients with paraphimosis should be referred to a urologist for consideration of circumcision.

MANAGEMENT

Phimosis – rarely needs emergency treatment. Balanitis may need treatment.

Paraphimosis –
1. Compress the glans firmly for five minutes to reduce oedema
2. Continue to compress the glans with your thumbs while drawing the foreskin forward over the glans with your fingers.

Plant ingestion

KEY POINTS

- Accurate identification of plant is essential
- National Poisons Information Service (NPIS) have plant identification system
- Everyday plants can be toxic.

ASSESSMENT

1. Assess ABC
2. Look for toxic syndromes, e.g. atropine-like effects of belladonna
3. Where was plant growing?
4. What type of plant?
5. Which part of plant was ingested, e.g. berry, leaves?
6. Identifying features of plant, e.g. colour, shape of flowers, berries, leaves.

INDICATORS OF NEED FOR FURTHER INVESTIGATION/ASSESSMENT

1. Toxic ingestions
2. Symptomatic patients

MANAGEMENT

1. Control airway, breathing and circulation
2. Consider naloxone if pinpoint pupils
3. Consider glucose if BM stix show hypoglycaemia
4. Consider atropine if sweating, salivation, muscle fasciculation, bradycardia
5. Supportive treatment
6. Identify plant in consultation with NPIS.

NONTOXIC PLANTS

1. Berries
   - berberis
   - cotoneaster
   - hawthorn
   - mahonia
   - mountain ash
   - pyracantha
   - skimmia
2. Flowers
   - antirrhinum
   - daffodil
   - bluebell
   - daisy
   - dandelion
   - fuchsia
   - geranium
   - orchid
   - rose
   - violet
3. Leaves
   - amalia
   - begonia
   - cacti
   - cheese plant
   - cyclamen
   - draconia
   - impatiens
   - rubber plant
   - spider plant
   - umbrella plant
   - yucca.

Retained earrings

Part of earring retained within the ear.

KEY POINTS

- Invariably lost stud into lobe of ear
- Same principles for lost rings in other areas
- Infection in ear lobe may be due to retained and forgotten stud
- Removal of stud is usually only treatment required for local ear lobe infection.

ASSESSMENT

1. Palpation usually confirms diagnosis
2. If not palpable, consider X-ray if metallic earring.

MANAGEMENT

1. Anaesthetize the posterior aspect of the ear lobe. Usually local infiltration with lignocaine is most appropriate. Topical EMLA is an alternative
2. Make a vertical incision on the posterior aspect of the ear lobe, passing through the piercing site
3. Clasp stud in pair of forceps and remove
4. If no evidence of infection, suture the wound
5. If infection present, leave wound open and apply dressing to ear lobe. Unless there is a spreading cellulitis there is no need for antibiotics.

AFTERCARE

1. Advise may need ear repiercing after wound fully healed
2. Not to use any earrings for at least three weeks or until fully healed for one week, whichever is longer.
3. Advise Afro-Caribbeans of risk of keloid formation.

Retained tampon

KEY POINT

Toxic shock is a life-threatening complication of a retained tampon.

ASSESSMENT

1. Careful and thorough speculum examination
2. Systemic assessment of patient including temperature.

INDICATORS OF NEED FOR FURTHER INVESTIGATION/ASSESSMENT

1. Systemic illness
2. Large amount of offensive discharge.

MANAGEMENT

1. Remove tampon under direct vision, ensure that it is all removed
2. Consider HVS and antibiotics if retained for more than 48 hours, or offensive discharge
3. Return/seek further help if continued discharge or systemic symptoms.

Ruptured long head of biceps

KEY POINT

Occurs spontaneously in the elderly.

ASSESSMENT

1. Bruising (may be extensive) around the elbow
2. Swelling appears in the upper arm
3. Assess for mobility at the elbow
4. Check distal neurovascular function.

INDICATORS OF NEED FOR FURTHER INVESTIGATION/ASSESSMENT

1. Suspicion of fracture
2. Inability to flex at the elbow.

MANAGEMENT

1. Provide analgesia
2. Advise exercise/refer to physiotherapy
3. Surgical repair is not usually required in the elderly if elbow flexion is still possible.

Safe accidental ingestions

KEY POINTS

- If in doubt check with local branch of Poisons Information Service (p. 143)
- Always check the container
- Drinking water or milk removes the taste.

THE FOLLOWING ARE SAFE:

Drugs
1. Antacids
2. Homeopathic drugs
3. Oral contraceptives
4. Vitamins, unless they include iron.

Household products
1. Soaps/detergents
   - bath oil
   - bubble bath
   - liquid soap
   - shampoo/shower gel
   - shaving foam
     (**NB** some washing powders and most dishwasher powders are hazardous)
2. Cosmetics/skin products
   - calamine
   - deodorant
   - hair conditioner
   - hand and body cream
   - lanolin
   - lipstick
   - mascara/eye liner
   - nappy cream

- petroleum jelly
- perfume/aftershave (but beware – alcohol content)
- suntan cream
- talcum powder
- toothpaste
- vaseline.

Other
- candles
- plasticine/clay
- sweetener tablets
- water base glues.

Not essential oils

NB See section on plant ingestion (p. 150).

Shingles

- Herpes zoster infection
- Immunosuppressed patients can have life-threatening infection
- Tingling sensation precedes blisters.

ASSESSMENT

1. Tingling sensation may start four to five days before rash appears
2. Check lesion is well localized
3. Should only affect one side of body and one dermatome
4. Check for evidence of immunosuppression
5. More common in elderly or debilitated
6. If involving face, check the eye.

INDICATORS OF NEED FOR FURTHER INVESTIGATION/ASSESSMENT

1. Pronounced fever, systemic illness
2. Other serious intercurrent disease
3. Eye involvement
4. Pregnant women.

MANAGEMENT

1. Leave rash exposed to dry it
2. Analgesia
3. Oral acyclovir if within 24–48 hours of rash appearing
4. Treat secondary infection.

Sinusitis

KEY POINT

Usually precipitated by acute viral upper respiratory infection.

ASSESSMENT

1. History of
   - frontal headache – worse on bending forward
   - headache between eyes, often described as 'splitting'
   - pain over maxillary sinuses
2. Examine for
   - features of URTI
   - tenderness over sinuses.

MANAGEMENT

1. Analgesia
2. Steam inhalations
3. Topical vasoconstrictors – short-term use only
4. Antibiotics – amoxycillin or erythromycin
5. Tetracycline (for exacerbated chronic sinusitis).

ADVICE TO PATIENTS

Recurrent acute attacks or severe chronic sinusitis may need ENT referral for definitive treatment.

INDICATIONS FOR REFERRAL

1. Doubts regarding the diagnosis
2. Suspicion of intracranial abscess
3. Neurological signs
4. Facial swelling.

Sore throat

Suspect glandular fever if not settling after one week.

ASSESSMENT

1. Check for size and appearance of tonsils
2. Check for lymphadenopathy
3. Check ears
4. Check ability to swallow.

REFER IF:

1. Unilateral tonsillar enlargement suggesting quinsy
2. Unable to swallow
3. Very sick/toxic.

MANAGEMENT

1. Simple analgesics and cold drinks give symptomatic relief
2. Most people do not require antibiotics
3. Antibiotics if:
   - tonsillitis
   - high temperature
   - painful lymphadenopathy
   - systemically unwell
4. Penicillin V is antibiotic of choice.

Subcutaneous abscesses

KEY POINTS

- Assess if appropriate for management in A&E
- Not appropriate if
  patient requires general anaesthetic, e.g. children
  abscess is too large for local anaesthetic
  abscess is likely to involve deeper spaces or structures,
  e.g. perianal abscess and web space abscess in hand.

ASSESSMENT

1. Check temperature
2. Blood sugar
3. Regional lymph nodes
4. Confirm need to drain abscess – painful, fluctuant, red
   swelling.

MANAGEMENT

1. Local anaesthesia – field block around the abscess
2. Incise along the length of the abscess
3. Express all pus and send sample for culture
4. Curette the entire cavity
5. Loose dressing to keep wound open
6. Review in two to three days
7. Antibiotic usually not indicated.

ALTERNATIVE

If the abscess is not considered ready for incision, give
antibiotics and review in two to three days.

Specific types of abscess

SEBACEOUS ABSCESS

1. May arise in a pre-existing cyst
2. Sebaceous material and fragments of cyst wall may be removed
3. Cyst may recur and can be dealt with electively if required.

HIDRADENITIS SUPPURATIVA

1. Recurrent abscess in areas of epocrine sweat glands, i.e. axilla, groin
2. Acute episode treated as for any abscess
3. Refer for definitive treatment.

PILONIDAL ABSCESS

Refer to general surgeons because of high risk of recurrence from simple drainage.

Sudden loss of vision

KEY POINT

This usually warrants an urgent referral.

ASSESSMENT

1. Likely presence of pain
2. Pattern of loss, e.g.
   - total loss of vision
   - 'curtain' across field of vision
3. Associated symptoms, e.g.
   - flashes of light
   - blurring
4. History of trauma
5. Examination
   - check pulse and blood pressure
   - visual acuity chart
   - ability to count fingers
   - ability to perceive light
   - if patient wears glasses, test when wearing glasses. If glasses are not available the patient must look through a pinhole in a card to minimize refraction error
   - visual fields
   - fundi.

NB Refer to ophthalmologist.

Sudden sensorineural hearing loss

KEY POINTS

- SUDDEN sensorineural hearing loss is an ENT emergency
- Most sensorineural loss is idiopathic, some is due to perilymph leakage, acoustic neuroma, syphilis
- Conductive loss is the differential diagnosis. It may be caused by ear canal obstruction, Eustachian tube obstruction, ear drum perforation (p. 149) or ossicle problems.

ASSESSMENT

1. History of onset, which side
2. Associated symptoms, e.g. vertigo, nausea, tinnitus
3. Look for discharge/bleeding from ear
4. Inspect ear canal and drum
5. Test with tuning fork:
   - Weber's Test. Place the vibrating fork on the forehead. This tests bone conduction, therefore the patient will state it is louder in the unaffected ear in sensorineural deafness, but in the deaf ear in conductive deafness
   - Rinné Test. Compare volume of fork held next to ear and held on mastoid process. In conductive deafness bone conduction is louder than air. In sensorineural deafness, it is the same as normal, i.e. air is louder than bone. A false result can be achieved by bone transmission to the normal ear.

INDICATORS OF NEED FOR FURTHER INVESTIGATION/ASSESSMENT

All cases of sensorineural loss should be referred urgently for treatment. Ask if specialist wants steroids given immediately.

Transient ischaemic attacks

KEY POINTS

- Sudden onset of loss of neurological function lasting less than 24 hours
- The majority last for minutes or a few hours
- Can affect any area of the brain, but most commonly cause hemiparesis, vertigo or aphasia
- See also sudden loss of vision (p. 162) and hearing (p. 163).

ASSESSMENT

1. Diagnosis is usually made on the history, as function has often returned by the time the patient seeks medical help
2. Ask about the onset and duration of the attack, including any associated symptoms such as palpitations or headache
3. Examine for precipitating causes, e.g. valvular heart disease, atrial fibrillation, carotid bruits, hypertension, diabetes
4. Full neurological examination for residual loss of function
5. Consider differential diagnoses such as fits, migraine, ocular problems, intracerebral bleeds.

INDICATORS OF NEED FOR FURTHER INVESTIGATION/ASSESSMENT

1. Headache is unusual with a TIA. Other causes such as haemorrhage or migraine should be excluded
2. Residual neurological symptoms or signs
3. Other precipitating or associated conditions requiring treatment, e.g. hypertension, arrhythmia.

MANAGEMENT

1. The management of TIAs is becoming more aggressive.

There are likely to be significant changes in the near future. Keep abreast of local policy developments and treat patients accordingly

2. If the episode has resolved completely and no other abnormalities have been detected, the patient may be discharged home. As a general rule patients should not be discharged alone after a TIA
3. Start aspirin providing not contraindicated
4. Arrange follow-up according to local policies
5. Advise the patient that they should return/seek help if the symptoms return or they feel unwell.

Urticaria

KEY POINTS

- A rash produced by degranulation of mast cells in response to a variety of stimuli. In many cases no cause is found but it may occur in response to cold, pressure, certain foods or drugs
- Usually short-lived with rapid onset, but can become chronic
- Can occur as part of the symptoms of anaphylaxis.

ASSESSMENT

1. Ask about onset, duration and precipitating factors
2. Ask about and look for symptoms and signs of anaphylaxis
3. The rash is red, raised and itchy.

INDICATORS OF NEED FOR FURTHER INVESTIGATION/ASSESSMENT

1. Presence of intraoral swelling, wheeze, tachycardia, hypotension, diarrhoea and abdominal pain are suggestive of anaphylaxis. This requires urgent treatment with oxygen, intramuscular adrenaline (intravenous if shocked), fluid resuscitation and monitoring
2. Patients with frequent episodes may benefit from further investigation by a dermatologist.

MANAGEMENT

1. Isolated urticaria without systemic signs or symptoms usually settles in a few days
2. Antihistamines will help to reduce itching

3. A short course of oral steroids can be used to stabilize mast cells and prevent further degranulation
4. Patients should be advised to return/seek help if they feel unwell, breathless or have worsening symptoms.

UTI/cystitis

KEY POINTS

- May present with a wide variety of symptoms
- Confirmation of UTI with a midstream urine is important for follow-up.

ASSESSMENT

1. Typical symptoms include dysuria, frequency of micturition, haematuria and suprapubic pain
2. Check temperature
3. Dipstick urine and send an MSU
4. Ask about previous UTIs and sexually transmitted diseases.

INDICATORS OF NEED FOR FURTHER INVESTIGATION/ASSESSMENT

1. Fever, loin pain and urinary symptoms are suggestive of pyelonephritis and should be investigated further
2. Proven UTI in a man or child and recurrent UTIs in women may need further investigation once the acute episode has settled
3. Gross haematuria is unusual with a simple UTI and needs further investigation.

MANAGEMENT

1. Advise the patient to drink plenty of fluids
2. Paracetamol or other simple analgesics for pain or discomfort
3. Send an MSU
4. Start antibiotics – usually trimethoprim or ampicillin initially.

ALTERNATIVES

Other acceptable forms of management include: If symptoms are not severe or are equivocal, send an MSU and advise patient to attend usual medical practitioner for treatment if required when the results are available.

Vertigo

KEY POINTS

- True vertigo must be distinguished from 'faintness', 'light-headedness' and 'dizziness'
- Subjective vertigo – impression of movement in space
- Objective vertigo – impression of objects moving around the patient.

ASSESSMENT

1. Pattern of attacks, e.g. duration, precipitating factors
2. Associated symptoms – headaches, tinnitus, hearing loss
3. Nystagmus
4. Positional testing.

MANAGEMENT

1. Benign positional vertigo (violent vertigo lasting <30 seconds and induced by certain head positions)
   - positional exercises
   - advice
   - vestibular sedative
2. Any vertigo not satisfying these criteria should be referred for further investigations.

REFERENCE

Lempert, T., Gresty, M. A. and Bronstein, A. M. (1995). Benign postural vertigo: Recognition and treatment. *BMJ*, 311, 489–491.

Managerial matters at minor injuries units

Confidentiality

KEY POINT

Medical information is confidential.

TELEPHONE INFORMATION

1. You do not know who is calling
2. Ideally let patient speak to caller
3. Ask patient before disclosing information
4. If in doubt, call the person back or do not give out details
5. Confine your comments to generalizations.

WHO MAY VIEW MEDICAL NOTES?

1. Only health care professionals involved in the treatment of the patient
2. All these people are bound by the same ethics of confidentiality.

NB Social services and employers do not have a right to view the records. Next of kin do not have an automatic right to medical information except for children.

WHEN CAN INFORMATION BE RELEASED WITHOUT THE PATIENT'S CONSENT

It can only be released to the police without consent when **all** the following apply:

1. It is in the public interest for the safety of others
2. Associated with a serious arrestable offence, e.g. rape, murder, manslaughter, child abuse
3. Senior doctor gives permission (consultant or GP)
4. Requested by senior police officer (inspector or above).

Traffic police investigating an accident may be told name, age and address of patient as well as brief description of injuries, severity and disposal of patient.

The court can order the release of medical records.

Discharge of elderly patient

KEY POINTS
- Always ensure patient is safe to go home
- Even a minor injury can tip the balance of a patient managing to cope
- Be careful leaving patient alone at night.

By answering the questions below the safety of discharging an elderly person should become apparent. The solution should also be evident.

ASSESSMENT

1. Is person safe to go home?
2. Have you seen person walking about safely?
3. What does person need to make them independent and is this available?
4. Who else is at home; how active are they?
5. Can person reach the toilet?
6. Who will provide meals?
7. Can person manage other daily activities?
8. Is condition liable to recur?
9. If happens again, will person be safe and will they be able to summon help?
10. Does person have a telephone or alert system to call for help?
11. Is medication understood?

MANAGEMENT

1. Are any relatives available to look after the person?
2. Can other members of community help, e.g. neighbours, church?

3. Can community medical care assist? District Nurse, bath service.
4. Can social services support be arranged? Home help, meals service, night service
5. Would a GP visit tomorrow be helpful?
6. Is hospital admission going to be required whilst problem is sorted out?

NB Only if you are still sure the person can manage safely at home should discharge be considered.

Documentation/ communication/follow-up

- Notes may be used by other health professionals, or by yourself later for reassessing the patient, writing reports etc.
- Record time, date, name at the start of your notes, time and sign on discharge
- Need to contain all relevant information, record important negatives as well as positives
- Diagrams are often helpful
- Note advice given to the patient, verbal and written
- Record follow-up advice – all patients should be told where to seek help if symptoms have not improved/get worse, e.g. GP, A&E etc.
- Ensure a letter or copy of the notes has been sent to whoever will be following up the patient.

NB Most complaints involve poor communication.

Violence and aggression

- Identifying and preventing violence and aggression is the best way to manage it
- Ensure your own safety at all times.

ASSESSMENT

1. Long waiting times, inadequate information and explanations and fear all contribute to violence and aggression
2. The following features suggest a situation is escalating – invading personal space, shouting or whispering, threatening gestures, pallor.

MANAGEMENT

1. Know how to call for help, e.g. alarm buttons, security, police
2. Do not get trapped. Avoid confined spaces, stay between the door and the aggressor
3. Make sure someone else knows where you are; if possible take someone with you
4. Try to remain calm and answer questions clearly and politely
5. Do not respond with anger or play to an audience
6. If you feel yourself becoming aggressive, stop and start again
7. If you feel unsafe, withdraw and call for help.

Index